Acknowledgements

This book is the culmination of a profound journey of spiritual discovery, introspection, and the integration of ancient wisdom with modern understanding. It would not have been possible without the support, inspiration, and guidance of many individuals.

First and foremost, I want to express my deepest gratitude to GOD, whose unwavering support and love have been my anchor through the highs and lows of life. Your belief in me and your encouragement have given me the strength to persevere and pursue my spiritual path with dedication.

I am grateful to the divine presence within and around us all, the source of all creation, for guiding me every step of the way. May this book be a reflection of the love, wisdom, and healing that is available to all who seek it.

To my family, friends and mentors, who have provided invaluable insights, wisdom, and encouragement throughout this journey—I am deeply thankful. Your conversations, whether challenging or comforting, have helped me refine my thoughts and deepen my understanding of the spiritual truths that form the foundation of this book.

I would also like to acknowledge the countless spiritual teachers, past and present, whose teachings have guided my spiritual growth. From the wisdom of the Bible to the insights of yogic traditions, your work has inspired me to explore the deeper connections between mind, body, and spirit.

Lastly, a special thank you to the readers, for whom this book is written. Your search for truth, healing, and spiritual fulfillment is what drives me to share my insights and experiences. I hope that the words in this book serve as a beacon of light on your own spiritual journey.

Thank you to everyone who has played a part in this journey. Your contributions, whether directly or indirectly, have helped bring this work to life.

Introduction

In a world inundated with information on health, spirituality, and self-improvement, this book stands apart as a unique synthesis of ancient wisdom and modern understanding. While many books explore the concepts of chakras, meditation, and spiritual health, few address the profound connections between these practices and the physiological realities of the human body, such as cerebrospinal fluid (CSF) circulation and the physical manifestations of our thoughts. This book does not merely scratch the surface; it delves deeply into the intricate relationships between the mind, body, and spirit, offering readers a comprehensive guide to achieving holistic well-being.

A Unique Approach to Spiritual and Physical Health

What sets this book apart is its integration of spiritual practices with scientific insights. It goes beyond the typical discussions of chakras and meditation by exploring how these practices influence and are influenced by the body's physical systems. The chapters on the alchemy of breath and CSF circulation, for example, provide a detailed examination of how controlled breathing and meditation can enhance neurological health and promote spiritual awakening. This fusion of ancient yogic practices with modern scientific understanding offers readers a new perspective on health that is both profound and practical.

Addressing Core Problems and Providing Solutions

This book addresses several key problems that many individuals face in their pursuit of health and spiritual growth:

Disconnected Practices: Many books and teachings treat spiritual practices and physical health as separate entities. This book bridges the gap, showing how practices like meditation and breathwork are not only spiritual tools but also critical for maintaining physical health, particularly in the brain and nervous system.

The Impact of Negative Thoughts: It tackles the often-overlooked issue of how persistent negative thoughts can manifest physically as disease, particularly cancer. By understanding the concept of "cancerous thoughts," readers are empowered to recognize and transform these destructive patterns before they manifest in the body.

The Role of Parasites in Spiritual Health: Unlike many spiritual texts that ignore the physical body's vulnerabilities, this book explores the connection between parasitic infections, chakra imbalances, and spiritual degradation. It provides practical advice on how to cleanse the body and spirit, ensuring that both are free from harmful influences.

Holistic Healing: Finally, this book offers a holistic approach to healing that integrates body, mind, and spirit. It provides readers with practical strategies for maintaining health through mindful breathing, proper alignment of the chakras, and awareness of how their thoughts and actions influence their overall well-being.

Why This Book is Essential

In a time when many are searching for deeper meaning and more effective ways to maintain their health, this book serves as a guide to achieving true holistic wellness. It does not offer quick fixes or superficial advice; instead, it provides a deep and thorough understanding of the interconnectedness of our physical and spiritual selves. Readers will find in these pages not only knowledge but also the tools to apply that knowledge in their daily lives, leading to lasting health and spiritual fulfillment.

This book is for those who are ready to go beyond the surface and explore the profound connections that shape our lives. It is a call to awaken to the power within, to take control of our thoughts and actions, and to live in harmony with the divine energy that flows through all things. Whether you are new to these concepts or have been on a spiritual path for years, this book offers fresh insights and practical guidance that will enrich your journey.

Chapter 1

Behavioral Manifestations of Parasitic Infections and Their Perception as Demonic Possession

Introduction: The Thin Line Between Physical and Metaphysical Explanations

Throughout history, human beings have struggled to explain behaviors and symptoms that defy the norms of what is considered natural or healthy. In many cultures, the physical ailments caused by parasitic infections have often been misinterpreted through a spiritual lens, leading to the belief that such symptoms are the result of demonic possession. This chapter delves into the specific behavioral changes caused by parasites, how these behaviors can be misinterpreted as signs of possession, and the broader implications of these perceptions. By exploring this complex interplay between the physical and metaphysical, we aim to provide a deeper understanding of how these ancient beliefs still resonate today.

Parasitic Infections and Behavioral Changes

Parasites are organisms that live on or inside a host, often causing harm in the process. When parasites invade the human body, they can lead to a range of physical and psychological symptoms, depending on the type of parasite and the area of the body it infects. Some of the behavioral changes caused by parasites include:

Neurological Disturbances: Certain parasites, such as Toxoplasma gondii and Taenia solium (which causes neurocysticercosis), can affect the brain, leading to seizures, hallucinations, and significant changes in personality. These symptoms can easily be mistaken for signs of possession, especially in societies where scientific explanations for these behaviors are not well understood. Additionally, these disturbances may induce experiences where individuals perceive the world through distorted, almost nightmarish lenses, which could be interpreted as mystical visions or spiritual encounters.

Extreme Fatigue and Weakness: Parasites like Plasmodium (responsible for malaria) and Trypanosoma (causing sleeping sickness) drain the body of energy, leading to extreme fatigue and weakness. This exhaustion can be seen as a loss of vitality or spiritual energy, reinforcing the belief that an individual is under the control of a malevolent force. The persistence of such *symptoms over time can also be associated with the metaphorical "fire that is not quenched," symbolizing a continuous drain on the individual's life force.*

Erratic or Violent Behavior: Some parasitic infections, such as those caused by Strongyloides stercoralis (threadworm) or Trichinella spiralis (which causes trichinosis), can lead to irritability, mood swings, and aggressive behavior. In extreme cases, the person may exhibit violent outbursts or self-destructive tendencies. Historically, these behaviors have been seen as clear indicators of demonic possession, especially when combined with other symptoms like sudden, unexplainable strength or the compulsion to harm oneself or others.

Historical and Cultural Interpretations

Throughout history, many cultures have struggled to understand the causes of unusual or extreme behavior. In the absence of scientific knowledge, these behaviors were often attributed to supernatural forces. This section explores how parasitic infections have been interpreted across different cultures and time periods:

Medieval Europe: During the Middle Ages, the concept of demonic possession was prevalent. Many individuals suffering from epilepsy, schizophrenia, or severe parasitic infections were believed to be possessed by demons. Exorcisms were performed in an attempt to rid the individual of the evil spirit, often leading to further psychological and physical harm. In some cases, the neurological effects of parasitic infections were likely responsible for the so-called "possession" symptoms, such as hallucinations or seizures, which were misunderstood due to the lack of medical knowledge.

African and Caribbean Traditions: In some African and Caribbean cultures, certain parasitic infections were believed to be the result of witchcraft or spiritual curses. The erratic behaviors caused by these infections were seen as evidence of possession by malevolent spirits. This belief was reinforced by the communal fear of contagion and the unknown, where physical symptoms were interpreted as spiritual manifestations.

Biblical Interpretations: The Bible contains numerous references to demons and evil spirits possessing individuals, causing them to exhibit strange behaviors. With modern understanding, some of these accounts could be reinterpreted as descriptions of parasitic infections or other medical conditions. For example, the "unclean spirits" that Jesus exorcized could be seen as metaphors for the parasitic or infectious diseases that plagued individuals, manifesting in behavioral and physical symptoms that were beyond the understanding of the time.

Case Studies and Anecdotal Evidence

To illustrate the connection between parasitic infections and perceived demonic possession, this section explores a few case studies and anecdotal accounts. These examples highlight how extreme behavior caused by parasitic infections has been misinterpreted as possession and the impact of these misinterpretations on the individuals involved:

Case Study 1: Neurocysticercosis in a Young Woman: A young woman in rural India began experiencing seizures and hallucinations. Her family believed she was possessed by a demon and sought the help of a local exorcist. After several failed exorcisms, she was finally taken to a hospital, where she was diagnosed with neurocysticercosis, a parasitic infection of the brain caused by the pork tapeworm Taenia solium. This case exemplifies how neurological disturbances caused by parasites can be misinterpreted as spiritual affliction, especially in regions with limited access to medical knowledge.

Case Study 2: Aggressive Behavior Linked to Strongyloidiasis: A man in a remote village in Africa began exhibiting violent behavior, attacking his family and neighbors without provocation.

The local community believed he was possessed by an evil spirit and performed several rituals to cleanse him. It was later discovered that he was suffering from strongyloidiasis, a parasitic infection that can cause severe neurological symptoms. This case demonstrates the thin line between physical illness and its spiritual interpretation, particularly in cultures where supernatural explanations are more accessible than medical ones.

Reinterpreting Spiritual Beliefs Through the Lens of Science

While it is essential to respect cultural and spiritual beliefs, it is also important to consider how scientific understanding can provide alternative explanations for behaviors traditionally attributed to supernatural causes. This section explores how parasitic infections can be reinterpreted through the lens of science, offering a more grounded explanation for symptoms that have historically been seen as demonic possession.

Modern Insights into Ancient Beliefs: By reinterpreting historical accounts of demonic possession through the understanding of parasitic infections, we gain a deeper appreciation for the complex interplay between physical health and spiritual beliefs. This reinterpretation does not diminish the spiritual experiences of those who believe in possession but rather offers a more compassionate and informed approach to understanding these experiences.

Balancing Science and Spirituality: This section emphasizes the importance of balancing spiritual beliefs with scientific knowledge. While spiritual practices like exorcism or cleansing rituals may provide comfort and psychological relief, they should be complemented by medical intervention when dealing with symptoms that could be caused by parasitic infections. By integrating both perspectives, we can approach the subject of parasitic infections and their effects on behavior with compassion, understanding, and a willingness to explore both the physical and metaphysical dimensions of health.

Conclusion:

The Intersection of Body and Spirit

This chapter concludes by emphasizing the complex relationship between physical health and spiritual beliefs. Parasitic infections, with their profound impact on behavior, serve as a poignant example of how easily the physical can be misinterpreted as the spiritual. By exploring these connections, we open the door to a more holistic understanding of health—one that respects both the body and the spirit. Through this understanding, we can provide more compassionate care to those who suffer from the effects of these infections, whether they manifest as physical symptoms or are perceived as spiritual afflictions.

Two Paths

In the heart of the bustling city of San Francisco, two young men, Jake and Tyler, faced the daunting task of making their way in the world, each grappling with his own deep-seated fears.

Jake, the older of the two by just a few months, had always been paralyzed by a fear of financial instability. His father had lost his job during the Great Recession, a trauma that left deep scars in Jake's understanding of what it meant to be secure. As a result, he stuck to safe choices, working a secure job in data entry, living in the same modest apartment for years, never risking a dime on his dreams.

Tyler, on the other hand, shared many of the same fears as Jake. He too had seen his family struggle, his mother juggling two jobs to make ends meet. But Tyler, unlike Jake, was determined not to let the fear of poverty define his life. He had aspirations of starting his own tech company, a dream fueled by his passion for coding and innovation.

One day, both men stumbled upon an opportunity. A local business incubator announced a competition for tech startups, promising seed funding and mentorship to the winner. Tyler saw it as a sign; he decided to quit his part-time job and dedicate himself fully to his startup idea. Jake, cautious as ever, decided not to participate, citing the financial risk and the slim chances of success.

Months passed, and Tyler worked tirelessly on his project. There were days of doubt and nights filled with fear of failure, but he pushed through, driven by a vision of what could be. His app, designed to help small businesses manage their finances more effectively, slowly took shape.

The day of the competition arrived, and Tyler, despite his nerves, pitched his heart out. The panel was impressed by his passion and the practicality of his app, awarding him the first place. The victory brought him not just the seed funding but also several offers of investment.

Meanwhile, Jake watched from the sidelines. He felt a mix of pride for his friend and a sinking feeling of regret. He saw in Tyler's success a lesson he wished he hadn't learned so late: the real risk was not in failing but in never trying.

Empowered by this realization, Jake finally decided to take a leap of faith. He enrolled in night classes for digital marketing, hoping to move away from the monotony of data entry and towards something that sparked his passion.

As years rolled by, Tyler's company grew, moving from a small startup to a significant player in the tech field. Jake, with his new skills, joined a startup himself, finding joy in the vibrancy of creative work.

In the end, both men conquered their fears, though in different ways and at different paces. Their journeys taught them that while the fear of survival might never entirely dissipate, facing it head-on was the only way to truly live. Their friendship, tested and strengthened by their individual paths, became a testament to the power of embracing one's fears and the possibilities that unfold when we dare to step beyond them.

Chapter 2

The Fire That Is Not Quenched: A Christ-Centered Approach to Fulfillment and Spiritual Healing

Introduction: Understanding the Spiritual Metaphor

This chapter explores the profound symbolism in the biblical passage from Mark 9:47-48, where Jesus speaks of "the fire that is not quenched" and "where the worm dieth not." Traditionally, this passage has been interpreted as a warning about the torments of hell. However, a deeper, Christ-centered approach reveals a more nuanced understanding that connects to spiritual fulfillment and healing. This new interpretation emphasizes how unfulfilled desires and unresolved attachments can lead to spiritual stagnation—a personal hell on earth.

The Spiritual Fire—A Metaphor for Unfulfilled Desires

The Fire That Is Not Quenched: In this reinterpretation, the "fire" represents the burning desires and ambitions that individuals carry throughout their lives. When these desires go unfulfilled—whether due to fear, shame, or societal pressures—they can consume a person, leading to a persistent feeling of emptiness and dissatisfaction. This inner fire, which is never quenched, symbolizes the ongoing torment of a life lived out of alignment with one's true self.

Chakra Connection: The Solar Plexus Chakra, often associated with personal power and desire, aligns with this interpretation. When blocked by feelings of shame or failure, this chakra can become a source of internal fire—an unquenchable hunger for fulfillment that is never satisfied. The fire here represents the burning need for recognition, success, or love that, when unmet, becomes a source of internal suffering.

The Worm That Dieth Not—Parasitic Attachments and Spiritual Stagnation

Worms as Symbols of Attachment: The phrase "where the worm dieth not" can be understood as a metaphor for the persistent attachments and unresolved emotions that continue to plague a person even after death. These "worms" are the remnants of unprocessed grief, guilt, or anger—emotional parasites that feed on the soul's energy, preventing it from moving forward.

Spiritual Interpretation: Just as physical parasites can drain the body of its vitality, these emotional worms drain the soul, keeping it trapped in a cycle of suffering and rebirth. This state can be seen as a form of hell on earth, where the soul is unable to find peace because it is continuously consumed by unresolved issues and unfulfilled desires.

Breaking the Cycle: To escape this cycle, one must confront and resolve these attachments. This involves deep spiritual work, such as forgiveness, self-compassion, and the pursuit of true desires. By addressing these issues head-on, individuals can cleanse their souls of these parasitic attachments, allowing them to move toward spiritual fulfillment and healing.

Jesus' Teachings as a Path to Liberation

Christ-Centered Fulfillment: Jesus' teachings encourage us to live in alignment with our divine purpose, free from the constraints of earthly desires and attachments. By following His path, we can avoid the internal fire of unfulfilled desires and the spiritual decay caused by unresolved attachments.

Practical Applications: This section provides practical advice on how to apply Christ's teachings to modern life. This includes daily practices of mindfulness, prayer, and meditation, all aimed at aligning one's life with spiritual principles and breaking free from the cycle of desire and attachment.

Mystical Insights—The Role of Parasites in Spiritual Visions

Visions of Hell Through a Parasitic Lens: Building on the concept of "the worm that dieth not," this section explores the idea that mystical experiences of hell could be influenced by the presence of parasites within the body. When a person enters deep meditative states, they may access visions that reflect the world through the perspective of these parasites—creatures that exist in a timeless, perpetual state of hunger and decay.

The Birth-Death Cycle and Spiritual Liberation: These visions can serve as a powerful reminder of the importance of spiritual purification. By cleansing the body of physical and spiritual parasites, one can break free from the birth-death cycle and achieve true liberation. This perspective encourages readers to approach their spiritual journey with a renewed sense of urgency and purpose.

Conclusion:

Embracing a Christ-Centered Path to Fulfillment

This chapter reinterprets the traditional warnings of hell as metaphors for the spiritual challenges we face in our daily lives. By understanding "the fire that is not quenched" and "the worm that dieth not" as symbols of unfulfilled desires and unresolved attachments, we can see how Jesus' teachings offer a path to true fulfillment and spiritual healing. Through Christ, we can overcome these challenges, cleanse our souls, and achieve a state of inner peace and spiritual liberation.

The Echoes of Forgiveness

In the bustling city of New York, two young women, Sarah and Emily, navigated the complexities of their lives, intertwined through years of friendship and shared experiences. They both worked in competitive fields—Sarah in digital marketing and Emily in law—and faced the pressures and pitfalls that come with striving for success in a relentless urban landscape.

Sarah, always the more introspective of the two, encountered a significant setback when a campaign she spearheaded failed dramatically. The blame fell heavily on her shoulders, and the wave of criticism from her peers was almost unbearable. Consumed by guilt and self-doubt, she spiraled into a pattern of self-criticism that clouded her days and haunted her nights.

Emily, witnessing Sarah's struggle, faced her own crisis when a high-stakes legal case she was managing went awry due to an oversight she had made. Unlike Sarah, Emily responded with defensiveness, externalizing the blame and insisting that the circumstances were beyond her control. She hardened her heart against any self-reproach and criticism, building a wall between herself and her colleagues, and even Sarah.

As the months passed, Sarah embarked on a journey of self-reflection. She attended workshops on emotional resilience and read extensively about the power of self-forgiveness. She learned that forgiving oneself was not a sign of weakness but of strength. It involved acknowledging her mistakes, learning from them, and understanding that one failure was not a definitive measure of her worth. Gradually, Sarah's perspective shifted; she began to reclaim her confidence, and her work improved. More importantly, she felt lighter, unburdened by the weight of her past actions.

Emily, meanwhile, noticed the change in Sarah but was unable to embrace a similar path. Her refusal to acknowledge her faults strained her relationships, both professionally and personally. She envied Sarah's newfound peace but remained trapped in a cycle of denial and bitterness.

The turning point came during an annual conference at which both women were invited to speak. Sarah shared her story of failure and forgiveness, speaking candidly about the importance of self-compassion in personal growth. Her authenticity resonated with many in the audience, earning her not only their respect but also their admiration.

Emily listened from the back, her emotions a tumult of denial and hidden despair. After the talk, she approached Sarah, and for the first time, she opened up about her own struggles. The conversation that followed was difficult but healing, with Sarah gently guiding her friend towards the path of self-forgiveness.

Months turned into years, and both women flourished in their careers and personal lives. Emily learned to embrace her vulnerabilities and found that in doing so, she was not only happier but more effective in her work. She repaired old relationships and built new ones, grounded in honesty and mutual respect.

Chapter 3

The Role of Chakras in Spiritual and Physical Health

Introduction:

Understanding Chakras

The concept of chakras originates from ancient Indian spiritual traditions, specifically from texts known as the Vedas, which date back over 3,000 years. The word "chakra" comes from the Sanskrit word for "wheel" or "disk," symbolizing the energy centers within the human body. Chakras are believed to be focal points of energy that correspond to various physical, emotional, and spiritual aspects of our being.

In Hinduism and later in Buddhism, chakras are considered vital to the flow of energy, or prana, through the body. There are seven main chakras aligned along the spine, from the base to the crown of the head. Each chakra is associated with specific bodily organs, emotional states, and spiritual functions. When these chakras are balanced, the individual experiences physical health, emotional stability, and spiritual clarity. Conversely, when they are blocked or imbalanced, it can lead to various physical and mental ailments.

What Are Chakras?

Chakras are considered to be spinning wheels of energy located within the subtle body, a non-physical counterpart to the physical body. The seven main chakras are believed to correspond to different areas of the body, influencing various organs, glands, and functions. These energy centers are not visible to the naked eye but are felt and experienced through spiritual practice and meditation.

Each chakra is represented by a specific color, mantra, and element, and it resonates with certain vibrations. The chakras are often depicted as lotus flowers, each with a different number of petals, symbolizing the levels of consciousness associated with them.

The Seven Main Chakras and Their Correspondences

Root Chakra (Muladhara)

Location: Base of the spine, pelvic floor

Color: Red

Element: Earth

Associated Organs: Adrenal glands, colon, bladder, lower digestive tract

Psychological Function: Grounding, survival instincts, safety, and security

Physical and Emotional Blockages: When the Root Chakra is blocked or imbalanced, an individual may experience anxiety, insecurity, or fear related to basic survival needs. This can manifest physically as digestive issues, lower back pain, or problems with the legs and feet.

Connection to Parasitic Infections: Parasites such as pinworms and tapeworms often reside in the lower digestive tract, an area governed by the Root Chakra. These parasites can drain physical energy, leading to fatigue and a sense of disconnection from the body.

Potential Cancers: Cancers associated with the Root Chakra include colon and rectal cancers, which affect the lower digestive system.

Sacral Chakra (Svadhisthana)

Location: Lower abdomen, just below the navel

Color: Orange

Element: Water

Associated Organs: Reproductive organs, kidneys, bladder

Psychological Function: Creativity, sexuality, pleasure, and emotional balance

Physical and Emotional Blockages: A blocked Sacral Chakra can result in issues related to sexuality, fertility, and emotional instability. It may also manifest as lower back pain, urinary tract infections, or reproductive issues.

Connection to Parasitic Infections: Parasites such as Trichomonas vaginalis, which affects the reproductive organs, can disrupt the balance of the Sacral Chakra. These infections can lead to physical discomfort and emotional disturbances related to intimacy and creativity.

Potential Cancers: Cancers associated with this chakra include cervical, ovarian, prostate, and bladder cancers, which affect the reproductive and urinary systems.

Solar Plexus Chakra (Manipura)

Location: Upper abdomen, stomach area

Color: Yellow

Element: Fire

Associated Organs: Stomach, liver, pancreas, small intestines

Psychological Function: Personal power, self-esteem, confidence, and willpower

Physical and Emotional Blockages: When the Solar Plexus Chakra is blocked, an individual may experience low self-esteem, lack of confidence, and difficulty making decisions. Physically, this can lead to digestive issues, ulcers, and problems with the liver or pancreas.

Connection to Parasitic Infections: Parasites like Giardia lamblia, which affects the small intestine, can disrupt the function of the Solar Plexus Chakra, leading to digestive problems and a feeling of powerlessness.

Potential Cancers: Cancers related to the Solar Plexus Chakra include stomach and liver cancers, which can severely impact digestion and metabolism.

Heart Chakra (Anahata)

Location: Center of the chest, near the heart

Color: Green

Element: Air

Associated Organs: Heart, lungs, thymus gland

Psychological Function: Love, compassion, empathy, and emotional balance

Physical and Emotional Blockages: A blocked Heart Chakra can result in difficulty forming or maintaining relationships, lack of compassion, and feelings of isolation. Physically, this may manifest as heart conditions, respiratory issues, or immune system problems.

Connection to Parasitic Infections: Parasites such as Toxoplasma gondii, which can affect the heart and lungs, are associated with the Heart Chakra. These infections can lead to respiratory issues, fatigue, and a diminished capacity for emotional connection.

Potential Cancers: Cancers associated with this chakra include breast and lung cancers, which directly impact the heart and respiratory system.

Throat Chakra (Vishuddha)

Location: Throat, neck area

Color: Blue

Element: Ether (Space)

Associated Organs: Thyroid, vocal cords, trachea

Psychological Function: Communication, self-expression, truth, and authenticity

Physical and Emotional Blockages: Blockages in the Throat Chakra can result in difficulty expressing oneself, fear of speaking the truth, or feeling misunderstood. Physically, this can lead to thyroid issues, sore throats, and problems with the neck and shoulders.

Connection to Parasitic Infections: Parasites like Ascaris (roundworm), which can migrate through the lungs and throat, are connected to the Throat Chakra. These infections can cause breathing difficulties and disrupt the ability to communicate effectively.

Potential Cancers: Throat and thyroid cancers are associated with this chakra, affecting the throat area and the ability to speak and communicate.

Third Eye Chakra (Ajna)

Location: Forehead, between the eyes

Color: Indigo

Element: Light

Associated Organs: Brain, pituitary gland, eyes

Psychological Function: Intuition, insight, imagination, and wisdom

Physical and Emotional Blockages: A blocked Third Eye Chakra can lead to confusion, lack of direction, and difficulty trusting one's intuition. Physically, this may manifest as headaches, vision problems, or issues related to the brain.

Connection to Parasitic Infections: Parasites like Toxoplasmosis, which can affect the brain and central nervous system, are linked to the Third Eye Chakra. These infections can cause cognitive impairments, vision problems, and disturbances in perception.

Potential Cancers: Brain cancers are associated with this chakra, impacting cognitive functions and mental clarity.

Crown Chakra (Sahasrara)

Location: Top of the head

Color: Violet or White

Element: Thought

Associated Organs: Brain, pineal gland

Psychological Function: Spiritual connection, enlightenment, and higher consciousness

Physical and Emotional Blockages: A blocked Crown Chakra can result in a feeling of disconnection from the divine, lack of purpose, and spiritual confusion. Physically, this may manifest as neurological disorders, migraines, or mental health issues.

Connection to Parasitic Infections: While direct parasitic infections in this area are rare, the overall health of the Crown Chakra is essential for maintaining spiritual well-being. Infections that affect the brain and nervous system can indirectly impact this chakra, leading to feelings of spiritual disconnection.

Potential Cancers: The Crown Chakra is not typically associated with specific cancers, but issues related to the brain and nervous system could be linked to this energy center.

The Interplay Between Chakras, Parasites, and Cancer

The relationship between chakras, parasites, and cancer is complex and multifaceted. While traditional medicine focuses on the biological aspects of disease, holistic approaches consider the energetic and spiritual dimensions as well. Parasites can disrupt the flow of energy within the chakras, leading to blockages that may manifest as physical ailments, including cancer.

Energy Flow and Disease: When the energy flow through the chakras is disrupted by parasites or other factors, it can lead to an imbalance that weakens the body's natural defenses. This imbalance can create an environment where diseases, including cancer, are more likely to develop.

Holistic Healing Approaches: Healing practices that focus on balancing the chakras, such as yoga, meditation, and energy healing, aim to restore the natural flow of energy and strengthen the body's ability to fight disease. By clearing blockages and ensuring the free flow of energy, these practices may help in the prevention and treatment of various ailments.

Parasites and Cancer Correlation: Some studies have suggested a link between chronic parasitic infections and the development of certain types of cancer. For example, the parasite Schistosoma haematobium has been linked to bladder cancer, while liver flukes (Opisthorchis viverrini and Clonorchis sinensis) have been associated with bile duct cancer. These infections may cause chronic inflammation, which can lead to cellular changes and increase the risk of cancer.

Historical and Cultural Perspectives on Chakras and Health

The concept of chakras is not confined to Indian traditions. Similar ideas about energy centers in the body have been found in various cultures around the world.

Chinese Medicine and Qi: In traditional Chinese medicine, the concept of qi (or chi) is central to understanding health. Qi is the life force that flows through meridians, which are similar to the chakra system in Indian traditions. Blockages or imbalances in the flow of qi are believed to lead to physical and emotional problems, much like the effects of blocked chakras.

Tibetan Buddhism: In Tibetan Buddhism, the chakras are known as "wheels of life" and are associated with specific spiritual practices aimed at achieving enlightenment. The flow of energy through the chakras is considered essential for spiritual awakening.

Western Adaptation: In the West, the concept of chakras was popularized in the 20th century through the work of spiritual teachers and practitioners who integrated Eastern philosophies with Western holistic practices. Today, chakras are commonly referenced in discussions of yoga, meditation, and alternative medicine.

Practical Applications for Chakra Healing and Prevention

Understanding the relationship between chakras, parasites, and health provides a foundation for practical healing approaches. By focusing on both physical and energetic health, individuals can take proactive steps to prevent and treat illness.

Chakra Meditation and Visualization: Practicing chakra meditation involves focusing on each chakra, visualizing it as a spinning wheel of energy, and using affirmations or mantras to clear blockages. This practice can help restore balance and promote healing.

Detoxification and Dietary Practices: Supporting the body's natural detoxification processes through diet and herbal remedies can help reduce the burden of parasites and improve overall health. Foods rich in antioxidants, fiber, and anti-parasitic properties (such as garlic, pumpkin seeds, and turmeric) can support both physical and energetic health.

Physical Exercises: Certain yoga poses are specifically designed to activate and balance the chakras. For example, the "Tree Pose" (Vrikshasana) is associated with grounding and stabilizing the Root Chakra, while the "Fish Pose" (Matsyasana) is linked to opening the Heart Chakra.

Integrative Health Practices: Combining traditional medical treatments with holistic practices offers a comprehensive approach to health. This integrative approach can include regular medical check-ups, parasite cleansing protocols, chakra balancing techniques, and mindfulness practices.

Case Studies and Anecdotal Evidence

To illustrate the connection between chakras, parasites, and health, this section will explore several case studies and anecdotal accounts. These examples demonstrate how individuals have successfully used chakra healing techniques to overcome physical and emotional challenges.

Case Study 1: Overcoming Chronic Fatigue Through Chakra Balancing: A woman suffering from chronic fatigue and digestive issues found relief after integrating chakra meditation into her daily routine. By focusing on the Root and Sacral Chakras, she was able to alleviate her symptoms and regain her energy.

Case Study 2: Healing Emotional Trauma Through Heart Chakra Work: A man dealing with unresolved grief and heart problems used a combination of Heart Chakra meditation, therapy, and lifestyle changes to heal both emotionally and physically.

Case Study 3: Preventing Cancer Recurrence Through Holistic Practices: An individual with a history of cancer in the reproductive organs used a holistic approach, including chakra balancing, detoxification, and dietary changes, to prevent the recurrence of the disease.

Conclusion:

The Integrative Approach to Spiritual and Physical Health

This chapter has explored the deep connections between the chakras, parasitic infections, potential cancers, and the corresponding areas of the body. By understanding the chakras as vital energy centers that influence physical, emotional, and spiritual health, we can take proactive steps to maintain balance and prevent disease. The interplay between traditional medicine and holistic practices offers a comprehensive approach to health, one that honors the body, mind, and spirit.

By embracing both ancient wisdom and modern science, individuals can navigate their health journeys with greater awareness and intention, ensuring that their chakras—and their lives— remain in harmonious balance.

The Story of James

A Journey from Letdowns to Triumph

James was a man in his early fifties, living in a small town where everyone knew each other's stories. His life, however, was not one he was proud to share. For years, James had been grappling with letdowns and disappointments, many of which he blamed on himself. He had tried his hand at various jobs, relationships, and personal projects, but nothing seemed to stick. Each endeavor ended in failure, leaving him with a deep sense of shame and self-doubt.

In his youth, James had dreams of becoming an artist. He spent hours painting, sketching, and imagining the life he would create for himself. But as the years passed, those dreams were slowly eroded by the realities of life. His first art exhibit was a disaster, attracting only a handful of attendees, none of whom bought any of his work. Feeling humiliated, James packed up his brushes and paints, telling himself that art was a childish pursuit and that it was time to grow up and find a "real" job.

He took on a series of odd jobs—construction, retail, delivery driving—each one more disheartening than the last. His relationships suffered too. James often found himself pulling away from those who cared about him, convinced that he was a failure and that he didn't deserve their love or support. His marriage, once full of hope and passion, crumbled under the weight of his unresolved disappointments. His wife left him, taking their two children with her, and James was left alone with his thoughts, which had grown increasingly dark and bitter.

As the years went by, James became more reclusive. He avoided social gatherings, afraid that others would see through the façade he put up—the façade of a man who was just fine, thank you very much. Inside, however, he was drowning in a sea of self-recrimination. He replayed his failures over and over in his mind, each time sinking deeper into despair. "If only I had been smarter, more talented, more disciplined," he would think, "maybe things would have turned out differently."

One cold winter evening, as James sat alone in his dimly lit apartment, he found himself staring at a blank canvas that had been collecting dust in the corner of his living room. It had been years since he had picked up a paintbrush, but something compelled him to take it up again. With a heavy heart and shaky hands, James began to paint.

At first, it was just to pass the time, to distract himself from the suffocating loneliness that had become his constant companion. But as the days turned into weeks, he found that painting brought him a sense of peace that he hadn't felt in years. The strokes of the brush, the blending of colors, the act of creating something from nothing—these were things that made him feel alive, if only for a little while.

One evening, as James finished a particularly emotional piece—a swirling, chaotic depiction of his inner turmoil—he sat back and looked at what he had created. For the first time in years, he didn't feel the familiar sting of shame or disappointment. Instead, he felt a strange sense of clarity. It was as if the act of painting had unlocked something within him, something that had been buried under layers of self-loathing and regret.

It was then that James realized the true reason for his failures: he had given up on himself. Each time life knocked him down, he had internalized the pain, allowing it to chip away at his self-worth. He had let the opinions of others define his value, and in doing so, he had lost sight of who he truly was. He had abandoned his passion, his gift, because he had been too afraid to fail again.

But now, as he stared at the canvas before him, James understood that failure was not the enemy. The real enemy was the fear of failure—the fear that had kept him from pursuing his dreams, that had driven him to settle for a life of mediocrity. He saw now that his failures were not signs of inadequacy, but opportunities for growth, lessons that had gone unheeded because he had been too blinded by shame to learn from them.

With this newfound insight, James made a decision. He would no longer live in the shadow of his past mistakes. He would embrace his failures, learn from them, and use them as stepping stones to success. He would paint, not for the approval of others, but for himself—for the joy and fulfillment it brought him.

James began to paint every day, pouring his heart and soul into his work. He revisited the dream he had once abandoned, and this time, he approached it with a sense of purpose and determination. Slowly but surely, his life began to change. His art gained recognition, not just in his small town, but beyond. Galleries began to take notice, and soon, James was hosting successful exhibits, each one more celebrated than the last.

But the real success, James realized, was not in the accolades or the sales. It was in the rediscovery of his passion, the reclaiming of his self-worth, and the knowledge that he had the power to shape his own destiny. He had learned that life's disappointments were not the end of the road, but rather detours on the path to fulfillment.

James had spent much of his life letting setbacks define him, but now he understood that it was never too late to start anew. His journey from failure to success was not just a story of personal triumph, but a testament to the resilience of the human spirit and the transformative power of self-belief.

Chapter 4

The Spiritual Significance of Blood and Purity

Introduction

The Essence of Life and Spiritual Purity

Blood has been revered across cultures and religions as the essence of life. In many spiritual traditions, it is seen not only as the carrier of physical vitality but also as a symbol of spiritual purity and divine connection. This chapter delves into the profound significance of blood in both spiritual and physical health, exploring its relationship with the concept of prana or life energy, the chakras, and the impact of parasitic infections and potential cancers. By understanding the spiritual and physical dimensions of blood, we can gain insights into the holistic nature of health and well-being.

Understanding Prana—The Life Energy

Prana, often translated as "life force" or "vital energy," is a concept deeply rooted in ancient Indian philosophy, particularly within the traditions of Hinduism, Buddhism, and yoga. Prana is believed to be the universal energy that flows through all living beings, sustaining life and connecting the physical, mental, and spiritual realms.

Origin of Prana: The concept of prana originates from the Vedic texts, dating back over 3,000 years. Prana is considered the breath of life, the cosmic energy that permeates the universe. It is said to flow through the nadis (energy channels) and chakras (energy centers) in the human body, maintaining health and vitality.

Prana and the Breath: In yoga and meditation practices, the breath is seen as the primary vehicle for prana. Techniques such as pranayama (breath control) are used to regulate the flow of prana, balance the chakras, and enhance spiritual awareness. The breath is not just a physical function but a means of accessing and directing life energy within the body.

Prana and the Blood: In the physical body, blood is considered the carrier of prana. It nourishes the organs, tissues, and cells, providing them with the energy needed to sustain life. The quality and flow of blood are seen as reflections of the state of one's prana. When blood is pure and circulates freely, it supports the harmonious flow of prana, leading to physical health and spiritual well-being.

The Role of Blood in Spiritual and Physical Purity

Blood is often associated with purity and sanctity in various religious and spiritual traditions. In Christianity, for example, the blood of Christ is symbolic of redemption and purification. In Hindu rituals, blood is considered sacred and is used in offerings and sacrifices.

Biblical Significance of Blood: The Bible frequently references the sanctity of blood as the essence of life. For example, Leviticus 17:11 states, "For the life of the flesh is in the blood, and I have given it to you upon the altar to make atonement for your souls; for it is the blood that makes atonement by the life." This passage highlights the belief that blood carries the life force and is central to spiritual purification.

Blood as a Carrier of Life and Spiritual Energy: In many cultures, blood is seen as the medium through which life energy flows. It is believed that maintaining the purity of blood is essential for both physical and spiritual health. Practices such as fasting, detoxification, and bloodletting were historically used to purify the blood and, by extension, the soul.

Blood and Karma: In some Eastern traditions, blood is also linked to the concept of karma. It is believed that the purity or impurity of one's blood reflects their karmic state. Actions that generate negative karma are thought to taint the blood, leading to physical and spiritual ailments.

Chakras, Blood, and Spiritual Health

The chakras, as energy centers, play a crucial role in the distribution of prana throughout the body. Each chakra is associated with specific organs and physiological functions, and the flow of blood is closely linked to the health of these energy centers.

Root Chakra (Muladhara) and Blood: The Root Chakra, located at the base of the spine, is associated with survival instincts, grounding, and physical vitality. It governs the adrenal glands and the lower digestive tract. The blood circulating through these areas carries the vital energy needed to maintain a sense of security and stability. Blockages in the Root Chakra can lead to issues such as poor circulation, anemia, and blood-related disorders.

Heart Chakra (Anahata) and Blood: The Heart Chakra, located in the center of the chest, is the seat of love, compassion, and emotional balance. It governs the heart, lungs, and circulatory system. The blood pumped through the heart is considered the physical manifestation of love and life force. When the Heart Chakra is balanced, the blood flows freely, supporting cardiovascular health and emotional well-being. However, blockages in this chakra can lead to heart disease, hypertension, and related conditions.

Solar Plexus Chakra (Manipura) and Blood: The Solar Plexus Chakra, located in the upper abdomen, is associated with personal power, self-esteem, and digestion. It governs the liver, pancreas, and small intestines, which are crucial for detoxifying the blood and maintaining its purity. Blockages in this chakra can lead to digestive issues, liver problems, and diabetes, all of which can affect the quality of the blood and overall vitality.

Parasites, Blood, and Spiritual Contamination

Parasitic infections can have a profound impact on both physical and spiritual health. Parasites are organisms that live on or inside a host, often causing harm by draining the host's resources, including blood. In spiritual terms, parasites can be seen as symbolic of negative energies or karmic impurities that contaminate the life force.

Impact of Parasitic Infections on Blood: Parasites such as malaria-causing Plasmodium directly infect the blood, leading to anemia, weakness, and other serious health conditions. These infections not only drain the physical body but also disrupt the flow of prana, leading to spiritual imbalances.

Spiritual Interpretation of Parasites: In many spiritual traditions, parasites are viewed as manifestations of negative karma or unresolved emotional issues. They are believed to thrive in environments where the life force is weak or blocked, feeding on the impurities in the blood and energy system. Clearing these parasites is seen as essential for restoring spiritual purity and physical health.

Parasitic Infections and Chakras: Each chakra governs specific areas of the body, and parasitic infections can disrupt the energy flow in these regions. For example, parasites in the digestive tract can affect the Solar Plexus Chakra, leading to issues with personal power and self-esteem.

Infections in the blood can impact the Heart Chakra, causing emotional disturbances and cardiovascular problems.

The Connection Between Parasitic Infections and Cancer

Recent studies have shown that chronic parasitic infections may increase the risk of certain cancers. This connection underscores the importance of maintaining both physical and spiritual purity to prevent disease.

Chronic Inflammation and Cancer: Parasitic infections often cause chronic inflammation, which can damage tissues and lead to cellular changes that increase the risk of cancer. For example, the parasite Schistosoma haematobium has been linked to bladder cancer, while liver flukes have been associated with bile duct cancer.

Energetic Imbalances and Cancer: From a spiritual perspective, cancer is seen as a manifestation of deep-seated energetic imbalances. These imbalances may be caused or exacerbated by parasitic infections, which disrupt the flow of prana and weaken the body's natural defenses. Healing these imbalances involves both physical treatments and spiritual practices aimed at restoring the flow of life energy.

Holistic Approaches to Cancer Prevention: Preventing cancer requires a holistic approach that includes both physical and spiritual practices. Detoxification, parasite cleansing, chakra balancing, and meditation are all essential components of a comprehensive strategy to maintain the purity of blood and prevent disease.

Case Studies and Anecdotal Evidence

This section explores case studies and anecdotal evidence that illustrate the connection between blood, prana, chakras, and health. These examples highlight the importance of maintaining purity in both the physical and spiritual dimensions.

Case Study 1: Overcoming Blood Disorders Through Pranic Healing: A man suffering from a severe blood disorder found relief through pranic healing techniques, which focused on cleansing the blood and balancing the chakras. His recovery demonstrates the power of combining spiritual practices with medical treatments.

Case Study 2: Parasite Cleansing and Emotional Healing: A woman with chronic fatigue and emotional instability underwent a parasite cleansing protocol combined with chakra meditation. As she cleared the parasites from her system, she also experienced a significant improvement in her emotional health and energy levels.

Case Study 3: Integrative Cancer Treatment and Chakra Work: An individual diagnosed with cancer in the reproductive organs used an integrative approach that included conventional medical treatments, dietary changes, and chakra work. By addressing both the physical and energetic aspects of her condition, she was able to achieve remission and maintain her health.

Conclusion: The Path to Spiritual and Physical Purity

This chapter has explored the deep connections between blood, prana, chakras, parasites, and health. Blood is not just a physical substance but a carrier of life energy that sustains both the body and the spirit. Maintaining the purity of blood through spiritual and physical practices is essential for overall well-being.

By understanding the spiritual significance of blood and the role of prana in maintaining health, we can take proactive steps to prevent disease and promote healing. This holistic approach to health honors the interconnectedness of the body, mind, and spirit, ensuring that we live in harmony with the divine life force that sustains us all.

Through the purification of blood and the balancing of chakras, individuals can restore the flow of prana and enhance their spiritual and physical health. By addressing parasitic infections, preventing energetic imbalances, and maintaining a healthy, pure lifestyle, we create an environment where both body and soul can thrive.

The Story of Emily

Finding Love Amidst Loss

Emily was a young woman in her late twenties, known for her vibrant spirit and warm heart. She had always been the kind of person who saw the good in everyone, who believed that life was full of possibilities. But life, as it often does, took a series of devastating turns that left her reeling.

It began with the sudden loss of her mother, a woman who had been Emily's anchor and best friend. The grief was overwhelming, a dark cloud that seemed to swallow up all the light in Emily's life. She found herself unable to find joy in the things that once brought her happiness. The days blurred into nights, and the nights into a restless kind of sleep, where dreams of her mother were shattered by the harsh reality of waking up to a world where she no longer existed.

Not long after, Emily's long-term relationship, which she had believed would end in marriage, crumbled under the weight of unspoken resentments and unmet expectations. The breakup left her heartbroken and questioning her worth. It was as if life was conspiring to strip away everything she held dear, leaving her adrift in a sea of loss and sadness.

Alone in her grief, Emily withdrew from the world. She stopped going out with friends, stopped engaging in the hobbies she once loved. Her apartment, once filled with laughter and light, became a place of solitude and silence. She couldn't understand how the world could go on turning when her own had come to a standstill.

One cold afternoon, as she sat by the window watching the rain trickle down the glass, Emily felt a sudden urge to go for a walk. It had been weeks since she had ventured outside, but something inside her—perhaps the faint whisper of her mother's voice—nudged her to get up and move. She wrapped herself in a warm coat and stepped out into the rain-soaked streets.

As she walked, the drizzle began to ease, and the clouds parted to reveal patches of blue sky. She found herself drawn to a nearby park, a place she had often visited with her mother. The trees, bare from the winter cold, stood like silent sentinels, their branches reaching out to the heavens. She wandered aimlessly, lost in thought, until she came upon a small, neglected garden tucked away in a quiet corner of the park.

The garden was overgrown, with weeds choking the life out of the few flowers that had managed to bloom. Yet, despite its disarray, there was something about the garden that caught Emily's attention. Perhaps it was the lone rose bush, still clinging to life amidst the decay, or the way the sunlight filtered through the trees, casting a golden glow on the weathered stone bench nearby.

Without thinking, Emily knelt down and began to pull at the weeds, her fingers digging into the cold, damp earth. She didn't know why she was doing it, only that it felt right. As she worked, a sense of calm began to settle over her, the physical labor providing a respite from the endless loop of sorrow that had been playing in her mind.

Days turned into weeks, and Emily returned to the garden every day. She cleared the weeds, pruned the bushes, and planted new flowers, watching as the garden slowly transformed before her eyes. It became a place of refuge, a sanctuary where she could be alone with her thoughts, yet feel connected to something greater than herself.

As the garden flourished, so did Emily's spirit. She began to see the world through new eyes, noticing the small acts of kindness that had always been there but had gone unnoticed in her grief. She saw the way a mother gently held her child's hand, the way the old couple on the bench shared a smile, the way the birds sang their songs of joy every morning.

One day, as she stood in the garden, now a vibrant tapestry of colors and life, Emily felt a warmth in her heart that she hadn't felt in a long time. It was then that she realized that love had been around her all along—in the beauty of the flowers, in the kindness of strangers, in the memories of her mother that lived on in her heart. Love was not something to be lost or found; it was everywhere, in every moment, in every breath.

Emily had found healing in the garden, but more importantly, she had found love—love for herself, for the world, and for the life that she had thought was irreparably broken. She understood now that while life could be filled with pain and loss, it was also filled with beauty and love. And it was this love that would carry her forward, guiding her through the darkest of times and helping her to bloom, just like the flowers in her garden.

With a renewed sense of purpose, Emily began to share her story, helping others who were struggling with their own grief and loss. She became a beacon of hope, showing that even in the darkest of times, love is always all around us, waiting to be found in the most unexpected places.

Chapter 5

Clearing the House: The Power of Love and Awareness in Transforming Inner Chatter

Introduction: Redefining the Metaphor of the "Clean House"

In the Gospels of Matthew and Luke, Jesus speaks of an "unclean spirit" that leaves a person and, finding no rest, returns to its former dwelling, now clean but empty. The spirit then brings with it more spirits, and the state of the person becomes worse than before. Traditionally, these passages have been interpreted with a sense of warning or caution—an image of doom and gloom. But what if we viewed them from a different perspective, one that emphasizes love, self-awareness, and the transformative power of conscious choice?

This chapter invites us to see these scriptures not as foreboding but as profound teachings about the power of our thoughts, the importance of cultivating positive habits, and the role of love in our lives. Once we become aware of our inner chatter—the continuous stream of thoughts that guide our emotions and actions—we gain the ability to choose whether to follow a positive or negative path.

The "Clean House" as a Metaphor for Inner Awareness

When Jesus speaks of a "clean house," we can interpret this as a mind that has become aware of its negative patterns and has made efforts to clear them out. This "house" is our inner world, our consciousness. By becoming aware of our destructive thoughts—what we might call "cancerous thoughts" in a previous chapter—we take the first step toward transformation. We "sweep" our inner house, recognizing the need to let go of harmful beliefs, grudges, fears, and habits.

However, clearing out the negative is only part of the journey. The critical next step is to fill that newly cleansed space with love, compassion, gratitude, and positive thoughts. If we neglect this step, we risk falling back into old patterns, often with even greater intensity. Just as Jesus warns that the "unclean spirit" may return with seven more spirits, so too can our negative habits and thoughts return stronger if we do not cultivate positive habits to replace them.

Recognizing the Inner Chatter: Choosing Love Over Fear

Inner chatter is the ongoing dialogue we have with ourselves—the thoughts that arise from past experiences, beliefs, and emotions. These thoughts can lead us in positive directions that promote growth, peace, and health, or in negative directions that reinforce pain, fear, and disease. The key is awareness. When we become conscious of our inner chatter, we are no longer at its mercy; we have the power to decide whether to continue down the same path or to forge a new one.

From a love-centered perspective, the "unclean spirit" represents our old negative habits, thoughts, or emotional patterns. These are not evil in themselves; they are simply patterns that no longer serve us. To replace them with new, healthier ones, we must recognize them, understand where they come from, and consciously choose to replace them with thoughts and habits grounded in love, kindness, and positivity.

The Physical Manifestation of Our Thoughts

As we explored in the chapter on "The Birth of Cancerous Thoughts and Their Physical Manifestation," our thoughts have a profound impact on our physical health. Negative thoughts can lead to chronic stress, inflammation, and ultimately, disease. Conversely, positive thoughts can promote healing, reduce stress, and enhance overall well-being.

The same principle applies here: if we cleanse our minds but do not fill them with love, gratitude, and joy, we may inadvertently allow negativity to take root once again, possibly with more force than before. This is why practices like meditation, prayer, gratitude journaling, and mindful breathing are crucial—they help "fill the house" with light, making it less hospitable to the "unclean spirits" of negativity and despair.

The Cycle of Returning to Old Habits

When we return to old habits after having made positive changes, those habits often come back stronger. This is because we have already experienced the benefits of positive change and are now consciously aware of the contrast. The awareness of what we are losing can make the old habit feel more intense or even harder to break. From a spiritual perspective, this is the moment when we must decide whether to let the "seven spirits" return or to stand firm in our commitment to positive change.

This is not about punishment or fear; it is about understanding the natural consequences of our choices. If we choose love, awareness, and positive habits, we fill our lives with light, reducing the likelihood of negativity taking hold. If we leave the house empty, we risk creating a vacuum that negativity can fill.

Practical Steps for Filling the House with Love

To truly transform our inner world, we need to fill it with practices and habits that align with love and positivity. Here are some practical steps:

- *Mindful Meditation and Breath Control: Regular meditation helps calm the mind and reduces inner chatter. Controlled breathing can help balance emotions and bring clarity.*
- *Gratitude Practice: Keeping a daily gratitude journal can shift your focus from what is lacking to what is abundant, filling your mind with positive thoughts.*
- *Positive Affirmations: Repeating affirmations that align with love and growth can help reprogram the subconscious mind and replace negative self-talk.*
- *Acts of Kindness: Engaging in acts of kindness, both toward yourself and others, creates a ripple effect of positivity and love.*
- *Spiritual Reflection: Whether through prayer, reading spiritual texts, or quiet reflection, connect with the divine within and around you, reinforcing the presence of love in your life.*

Conclusion: A Journey of Continuous Cleansing and Filling

In life, there will always be opportunities to cleanse our inner world and start anew. But the true work lies in continuously filling that space with light, love, and positive energy. By consciously choosing what we allow to take up residence in our "house," we empower ourselves to live a life of purpose, fulfillment, and spiritual growth.

Remember, it is not enough to clear away the darkness; we must also light the candle of love within us and keep it burning bright. Only then can we truly transform from within, ensuring that our "house" remains a place of peace, joy, and divine connection.

The Story of Sarah and Lily

The Power of Inner Chatter

Sarah and Lily were colleagues at a bustling marketing firm, known for its high-pressure environment and demanding deadlines. Both women were equally talented and dedicated to their work, but they approached life with very different mindsets.

Sarah was known for her positive and uplifting inner chatter. She had a habit of encouraging herself, even in the face of challenges. Her thoughts were filled with affirmations like, "I can do this," and "Every problem has a solution." No matter how tough things got, Sarah managed to stay calm and focused, always finding a way to navigate through the storm with grace and optimism.

Lily, on the other hand, struggled with negative inner chatter. Her mind was a constant battleground of self-criticism and doubt. "I'm not good enough," she would think when faced with a difficult task. "I always mess things up," she would tell herself after making a mistake. Lily's thoughts were harsh and unforgiving, and over time, they began to take a toll on her confidence and well-being.

At work, Sarah and Lily's differences in mindset became increasingly apparent. While Sarah seemed to thrive under pressure, Lily often felt overwhelmed and defeated. She admired Sarah's ability to stay positive, but she couldn't understand how Sarah managed to maintain such a mindset, especially when things didn't go as planned.

One particularly stressful day, the team was given an urgent project with an impossible deadline. As the pressure mounted, Lily's negative inner chatter became more intense. "There's no way I can do this," she thought. "I'm going to fail, and everyone will see how incompetent I am." The more she thought this way, the more anxious and paralyzed she became.

Meanwhile, Sarah was facing the same challenges but with a different internal dialogue. She told herself, "This is tough, but I've handled tough situations before. I'll take it one step at a time and do my best." Her calm, positive inner chatter helped her stay focused and productive, even as the deadline loomed.

That evening, after a particularly rough day, Lily found herself alone in the office, staring at her computer screen. She had fallen behind on the project, and her thoughts were spiraling out of control. "Why am I so bad at this? Why can't I be more like Sarah?" she muttered to herself, feeling the familiar sting of self-doubt.

But then, something shifted. For the first time, Lily became fully aware of the harshness of her inner chatter. She caught herself thinking, "I'm terrible at this," and realized just how destructive that thought was. She paused and reflected on how she had been talking to herself all these years. It dawned on her that her inner chatter was not just unhelpful—it was sabotaging her success and happiness.

Lily remembered how Sarah always seemed to stay positive, no matter what. "Maybe," she thought, "it's not that Sarah is better at handling stress, but that she talks to herself differently."

With this newfound awareness, Lily decided to try something different. She took a deep breath and began to challenge her negative thoughts. Instead of saying, "I'm going to fail," she told herself, "I'm doing the best I can, and that's enough." Instead of thinking, "I always mess things up," she said, "I've made mistakes, but I've learned from them."

At first, it felt strange and unnatural, but Lily persisted. She realized that just as she had conditioned herself to think negatively, she could recondition her mind to think more positively. Slowly but surely, her inner chatter began to change.

Over the next few weeks, Lily noticed a remarkable difference. She felt less anxious and more confident in her abilities. She was more productive at work and found herself enjoying her tasks rather than dreading them. The more she practiced positive self-talk, the more natural it became, and the more her outlook on life improved.

One day, as she and Sarah were grabbing coffee, Lily confided in her colleague about the changes she had been making. "I used to be so hard on myself," Lily admitted, "but I've started to realize that how I talk to myself makes all the difference."

Sarah smiled warmly. "It's amazing how much power our thoughts have," she said. "Once you start speaking to yourself with kindness and encouragement, everything else falls into place."

Lily nodded, grateful for the insight and for the transformation that had begun within her. She had learned a tough lesson, but one that had set her on a path to a more fulfilling and successful life.

In the end, Lily realized that the key to her happiness and success wasn't in external achievements or the approval of others—it was in the way she spoke to herself. By changing her inner chatter, she had unlocked the door to a more positive and empowered life, one where she could truly thrive.

Chapter 6

Spiritual Warfare – Purging Parasitic Demons and Cancerous Thoughts

Introduction: The Battle Between Light and Darkness

The concept of spiritual warfare is deeply rooted in many religious and spiritual traditions, symbolizing the eternal struggle between good and evil, light and darkness. In this context, demons are often viewed as malevolent forces that seek to corrupt the soul and disrupt the balance of the body, mind, and spirit. However, in recent times, this idea has expanded to include a more metaphorical understanding of demons—specifically, the negative thoughts, emotions, and behaviors that can consume an individual from within.

This chapter delves into the complex relationship between spiritual warfare, parasitic infections, and the chakras, exploring how these forces interact to influence physical, mental, and spiritual health. By understanding the origins and characteristics of demons, the behaviors associated with possession, and the effects of parasitic infections on the body, we can develop strategies for purging these destructive influences and restoring harmony to our lives.

Understanding Demons and Their Origins

Demons have been described in various religious texts and spiritual traditions as malevolent entities that seek to harm humans by possessing their bodies and corrupting their souls. The idea of demonic possession has been a part of human culture for millennia, with roots in ancient Mesopotamian, Egyptian, Greek, and Roman beliefs. In Christianity, demons are often depicted as fallen angels who rebelled against God and now seek to lead humanity astray.

Biblical Perspective: In the Bible, demons are frequently associated with evil spirits that possess individuals, causing them to exhibit strange and often harmful behaviors. For example, in the New Testament, Jesus is depicted as casting out demons from those who were afflicted, restoring them to health and sanity. This connection between demons and physical or mental illness has influenced the way many cultures interpret unusual or extreme behaviors.

Cultural Interpretations: Different cultures have their interpretations of demons and possession. In some African and Caribbean traditions, demons are believed to be spirits of the dead or malevolent entities sent by witches to harm others. In these contexts, possession is often seen as a form of spiritual attack, requiring intervention through rituals, exorcisms, or other forms of spiritual cleansing.

Metaphorical Demons: In modern spiritual practices, demons are also understood metaphorically as the negative thoughts, emotions, and behaviors that can take hold of a person and lead them down a destructive path. These "demons" can manifest as fear, anger, guilt, shame, and other negative states that disrupt the balance of the chakras and weaken the flow of prana (life energy) in the body.

Characteristics of Demonic Possession and Parasitic Infections

Demonic possession has traditionally been described as a state in which an individual is controlled by a malevolent entity, leading to behaviors and symptoms that are often beyond the person's control. Similarly, parasitic infections can take over the body, causing physical and mental changes that mirror the symptoms of possession.

Symptoms of Possession: Common symptoms of demonic possession include sudden personality changes, violent outbursts, self-harm, speaking in unknown languages, and exhibiting superhuman strength. These symptoms are often accompanied by a sense of inner torment, as if the individual is being controlled by an external force.

Behavioral Changes Due to Parasitic Infections: Parasitic infections can cause a range of physical and psychological symptoms that may be mistaken for signs of possession. For example, neurocysticercosis, caused by the pork tapeworm Taenia solium, can lead to seizures, hallucinations, and personality changes. Similarly, Toxoplasma gondii can affect the brain, leading to behavioral changes, increased risk-taking, and other psychological effects.

Overlap Between Possession and Parasitic Infections: The similarities between the symptoms of demonic possession and parasitic infections suggest that some historical accounts of possession may have been misinterpretations of parasitic diseases. For example, the convulsions and hallucinations associated with certain parasitic infections could easily be seen as evidence of possession in cultures without a scientific understanding of these conditions.

Chakras, Parasites, and the Spiritual Body

The chakras are energy centers within the body that correspond to different aspects of physical, emotional, and spiritual health. When these energy centers are balanced and functioning *properly, they allow the free flow of prana, leading to a state of overall well-being. However, when the chakras are blocked or imbalanced—whether by negative thoughts, emotions, or parasitic infections—the flow of prana is disrupted, leading to physical and spiritual ailments.*

Root Chakra (Muladhara): The Root Chakra, located at the base of the spine, is associated with grounding, survival, and physical vitality. Parasitic infections in the lower digestive tract, such as those caused by pinworms or tapeworms, can disrupt this chakra, leading to feelings of insecurity, fear, and a lack of grounding. In spiritual terms, these infections may be seen as manifestations of "demons" that feed on fear and survival instincts.

Sacral Chakra (Svadhisthana): The Sacral Chakra, located in the lower abdomen, governs creativity, sexuality, and emotional balance. Infections in the reproductive organs, such as those caused by Trichomonas vaginalis, can lead to imbalances in this chakra, manifesting as issues related to guilt, shame, and sexual dysfunction. These "demons" of guilt and shame can prevent individuals from fully expressing their creative and emotional potential.

Solar Plexus Chakra (Manipura): The Solar Plexus Chakra, located in the upper abdomen, is associated with personal power, self-esteem, and digestion. Parasitic infections in the digestive system, such as giardiasis, can lead to imbalances in this chakra, resulting in feelings of powerlessness, low self-esteem, and digestive issues. The "demons" of doubt and lack of self-worth can undermine an individual's sense of personal power and confidence.

Heart Chakra (Anahata): The Heart Chakra, located in the center of the chest, is the seat of love, compassion, and emotional balance. Infections affecting the heart and lungs, such as those caused by lung flukes, can disrupt this chakra, leading to feelings of grief, sadness, and isolation. The "demons" of grief and loss can close off the heart, preventing individuals from experiencing love and connection.

Throat Chakra (Vishuddha): The Throat Chakra, located in the throat area, governs communication, self-expression, and truth. Parasitic infections affecting the respiratory system, such as roundworm infections, can block this chakra, leading to difficulties in communication and self-expression. The "demons" of lies and suppressed truth can stifle one's voice and ability to speak authentically.

Third Eye Chakra (Ajna): The Third Eye Chakra, located between the eyebrows, is associated with intuition, insight, and spiritual vision. Parasitic infections affecting the brain, such as toxoplasmosis, can cloud this chakra, leading to confusion, lack of direction, and difficulty accessing intuition. The "demons" of illusion and deception can obscure one's inner vision and spiritual insight.

Crown Chakra (Sahasrara): The Crown Chakra, located at the top of the head, is the center of spiritual connection, enlightenment, and divine consciousness. Although direct parasitic infections in this area are rare, any disruption in the overall energy system can impact this chakra, leading to a sense of disconnection from the divine and a lack of spiritual purpose. The "demons" of earthly attachment and materialism can prevent individuals from experiencing true spiritual fulfillment.

Purging Parasitic Demons and Cancerous Thoughts

Purging parasitic demons and cancerous thoughts requires a multifaceted approach that addresses both the physical and spiritual dimensions of health. By understanding the interconnectedness of the body, mind, and spirit, individuals can develop strategies for cleansing their energy systems and restoring balance.

Physical Cleansing: The first step in purging parasitic demons is to address any physical infections in the body. This may involve medical treatments, such as antiparasitic medications, as well as natural remedies, such as herbal cleanses and detoxification protocols. Maintaining a healthy diet, rich in anti-parasitic foods like garlic, pumpkin seeds, and turmeric, can also support the body's natural defenses against parasites.

Spiritual Cleansing: In addition to physical cleansing, spiritual practices are essential for purging negative energies and restoring the flow of prana. Chakra meditation, energy healing, and visualization techniques can help to clear blockages and balance the chakras. Pranayama (breath control) exercises can also be used to regulate the flow of prana and strengthen the connection between the body and spirit.

Mindful Awareness: Purging cancerous thoughts requires cultivating mindful awareness of one's mental and emotional states. By observing and acknowledging negative thoughts and emotions, individuals can begin to release them and replace them with positive, life-affirming beliefs. Practices such as journaling, affirmations, and mindfulness meditation can support this process.

Faith and Spiritual Practice: For those who follow a religious or spiritual path, faith can be a powerful tool in the battle against parasitic demons. Prayer, scripture study, and participation in spiritual rituals can provide strength, guidance, and protection against negative influences. Calling upon divine assistance, whether through prayer or invocation, can help to dispel dark energies and restore spiritual purity.

Case Studies and Anecdotal Evidence

To illustrate the effectiveness of these practices, this section will explore several case studies and anecdotal accounts of individuals who have successfully purged parasitic demons and cancerous thoughts from their lives. These examples demonstrate the power of combining physical, mental, and spiritual approaches to achieve holistic healing.

Case Study 1: Healing from Neurocysticercosis: A young woman suffering from neurocysticercosis, which caused seizures and severe personality changes, was initially thought to be possessed. After receiving appropriate medical treatment to eliminate the parasite from her brain, she also engaged in chakra balancing meditation and energy healing to restore her mental and emotional health. This integrative approach helped her regain a sense of peace and stability.

Case Study 2: Overcoming Chronic Anxiety Through Parasite Cleansing and Spiritual Practice: A middle-aged man with a long history of anxiety and gastrointestinal issues discovered that he was suffering from a parasitic infection. After undergoing a parasite cleanse and incorporating daily spiritual practices, including prayer and chakra meditation, his symptoms significantly improved. He reported feeling more grounded, secure, and spiritually connected.

Case Study 3: Cancer Remission and Chakra Balancing: A woman diagnosed with breast cancer attributed her healing to a combination of conventional medical treatments and holistic practices, including chakra balancing and parasite cleansing. She believed that addressing both the physical tumor and the underlying energetic imbalances allowed her to achieve remission and maintain her health.

Conclusion:

The Path to Spiritual Warfare and Healing

This chapter has explored the profound connections between chakras, parasitic infections, potential cancers, and the concept of demonic possession. By understanding demons not only *as malevolent entities but also as metaphorical representations of negative thoughts, emotions, and behaviors, we can see how these "demons" disrupt the balance of our energy systems and lead to physical and spiritual ailments.*

The practice of spiritual warfare, in this context, involves purging these parasitic demons and cancerous thoughts through a combination of physical cleansing, spiritual practices, and mindful awareness. By addressing the interconnectedness of the body, mind, and spirit, individuals can reclaim their power, restore balance, and achieve holistic health.

As we navigate the complexities of modern life, it is essential to remain vigilant in maintaining our spiritual purity and protecting ourselves from the negative forces that seek to disrupt our well-being. Whether these forces manifest as actual parasitic infections or metaphorical demons, the principles of spiritual warfare provide us with the tools and strategies needed to overcome them and live in harmony with our divine purpose.

Chapter 7

Awakening to Inner Truth: Transforming Toxic Patterns Through Awareness and Compassion

Introduction: The Journey from Blindness to Awareness

In our journey toward spiritual and physical well-being, one of the greatest challenges is recognizing the parts of our lives that cause us harm. Often, these harmful patterns are so ingrained in our daily routines, thoughts, and environments that they become almost invisible to us. This chapter is an invitation to open our eyes, to see clearly the patterns that keep us stuck, and to embrace a new way of being through awareness, love, and intentional action.

The aim is not to force change upon anyone but to gently guide each individual, helping them see their lives from a higher perspective and empowering them to choose love over fear, clarity over confusion, and growth over stagnation.

Recognizing the Patterns: The First Step Toward Transformation

Awareness is the first and most crucial step in transformation. Before we can make meaningful changes in our lives, we must first recognize what needs to change. This involves a process of self-reflection and honest assessment, where we look at our thoughts, reactions, and environments with fresh eyes.

- *Identifying Toxic Triggers: Encourage yourself to look at your day-to-day experiences and pinpoint moments where you feel disconnected, angry, fearful, or upset. What thoughts, environments, or interactions trigger these feelings? Understand that identifying these triggers is not about judgment; it is about awareness.*
- *Seeing the Patterns Without Judgment: Approach this process with self-compassion. Understand that everyone has blind spots and that recognizing these patterns is the beginning of freedom, not a reason for self-criticism.*

Inner Chatter: Observing Without Attachment

The inner chatter is the continuous dialogue we have with ourselves, often influenced by past experiences, fears, and insecurities. Learning to observe this chatter without attachment is key to shifting from negative to positive thought patterns.

- *The Concept of "Inner Weather": Thoughts and emotions can be seen as "inner weather"—they come and go, and we do not have to react to every storm that arises. By observing our thoughts without becoming entangled in them, we create a gap between the experience and our reaction.*
- *The Power of Choice: Once we recognize these patterns, we have the power to choose whether to let them lead us in a positive or negative direction. The truth is, negative habits or ways of thinking that once served us may no longer be beneficial. Letting go is a sign of growth, not weakness.*

The Role of Meditation: Anchoring in the Eye of the Storm

Meditation is not just a practice; it is a tool for reconnection and grounding. The meditation method shared in this book is designed to help anchor oneself in a state of peace and clarity, especially when surrounded by a toxic environment.

- *Daily Practice with Intention: The effectiveness of meditation lies in consistency and intention. Approach each session with the goal of reconnecting with your inner peace, not just as an escape from external chaos.*
- *Using Meditation to Rebuild After Disconnect: Understand that it is natural to feel disconnected when returning to a toxic environment. Meditation is your home base; returning to it regularly helps reinforce your connection and reduces the influence of negative surroundings.*

Building the Foundation for Positive Change

To ensure that the transformative effects of awareness and meditation are sustained, it is crucial to cultivate positive habits and create a supportive environment, both internally and externally.

- *Personal Peace Plans: Create a personalized "peace plan" that includes specific affirmations, breathwork, visualizations, and grounding exercises tailored to your unique challenges. This serves as a toolkit for moments of disconnect.*
- *Creating Sacred Spaces: Even within toxic environments, having a dedicated sacred space for meditation and reflection can provide a much-needed anchor. This space could be as simple as a corner with calming objects or as elaborate as a dedicated room.*

Practical Steps for Cultivating Awareness and Letting Go

Real transformation comes from combining awareness with action. Here are practical steps to help you cultivate awareness and let go of what no longer serves you:

- *Mindful Reflection and Self-Inquiry: Practice asking yourself, "Is holding onto this thought or reaction helping me? What would happen if I let it go?" This process of inquiry helps you see how attachment to certain thoughts may be causing more harm than good.*
- *Self-Compassion Practices: Treat yourself with kindness, especially when confronting old habits or patterns. Remember, letting go is a process, and growth is not linear. Celebrate the small wins along the way.*
- *Reframing Challenges as Opportunities for Growth: Each moment of disconnection or challenge is an opportunity to practice reconnecting to your inner truth. Reframe these experiences as valuable lessons rather than failures.*

Encouraging Sustainable Change: From Knowledge to Wisdom

Knowledge is knowing what needs to change; wisdom is the practice of changing it. Encourage yourself to go beyond intellectual understanding and put these teachings into daily practice. Understand that sustainable change comes from consistency, commitment, and an unwavering belief in your capacity to grow and transform.

- *Create a Support System: Connect with like-minded individuals who support your journey and hold space for your growth. This can be a meditation group, an online community, or a trusted friend.*
- *Regular Check-Ins and Accountability: Consistent reflection on your progress helps to keep you on track and allows you to make necessary adjustments to your practice or mindset.*

Conclusion: A Continuous Journey of Self-Discovery and Compassion

This chapter is a reminder that transformation is not a destination but a continuous journey of self-discovery and compassion. By recognizing the parts of your life that hurt you and consciously choosing to change how you think about and react to them, you are reclaiming your power. You are not a victim of your circumstances but a creator of your reality.

Meditation, mindfulness, and self-awareness are your tools; love, compassion, and patience are your guides. With these, you can navigate even the most toxic environments and emerge stronger, more connected, and more at peace with yourself and the world around you.

Chapter 8

The Birth of Cancerous Thoughts and Their Physical Manifestation

Introduction: The Power of Thoughts in Shaping Reality

Thoughts are powerful forces that shape our reality. They influence our emotions, behaviors, and ultimately our physical health. While positive thoughts can promote well-being and healing, negative thoughts can be deeply destructive, leading to what can be described as "cancerous thoughts." These are persistent, heavy, and negative mental patterns that can fester within the mind, affecting not only mental and emotional health but also manifesting physically in the body as diseases, including cancer.

This chapter explores the origins and nature of cancerous thoughts, their connection to the chakras, and how they can lead to physical manifestations such as cancer. We will also delve into the role of parasites in exacerbating these thoughts and their potential to disrupt the body's energy systems.

Understanding Cancerous Thoughts

Cancerous thoughts are negative, persistent thought patterns that, like a malignancy in the body, grow and spread if not addressed. These thoughts can stem from various sources, including trauma, fear, guilt, shame, and unresolved emotional issues. They are "cancerous" in the sense that they consume the mental and emotional energy of an individual, leading to spiritual, emotional, and eventually physical decay.

Origins of Cancerous Thoughts: The idea of thoughts affecting physical health is not new. Ancient philosophies, such as those found in Eastern traditions, have long held that the mind and body are interconnected. In modern psychology, the concept of cognitive-behavioral patterns highlights how negative thoughts can lead to negative emotions and behaviors, creating a cycle that is difficult to break.

The Process of Thought Manifestation: Thoughts are energy, and when they are repeated and focused upon, they become more potent. Negative thoughts, particularly those that are deeply rooted in fear, guilt, or shame, can create energetic blockages in the body's energy system, specifically in the chakras. Over time, these blockages can manifest as physical ailments, including cancer.

The Birth of Cancerous Thoughts: These thoughts often begin as small, seemingly insignificant worries or fears. However, when they are not addressed or resolved, they grow and accumulate, much like cancer cells. As these thoughts persist, they begin to affect the individual's overall energy field, creating a fertile ground for disease.

Chakras and the Energy System

The chakras are the body's energy centers, each corresponding to different aspects of physical, emotional, and spiritual health. When the chakras are balanced and healthy, they allow the free flow of prana (life energy) throughout the body, promoting well-being. However, when they are blocked or imbalanced—often due to cancerous thoughts—the flow of energy is disrupted, leading to physical and emotional problems.

Root Chakra (Muladhara): The Root Chakra, located at the base of the spine, is associated with survival instincts, grounding, and physical vitality. Cancerous thoughts related to fear and insecurity can block this chakra, leading to issues such as chronic stress, anxiety, and disorders of the lower digestive system. Physically, this can manifest as colon or rectal cancer.

Sacral Chakra (Svadhisthana): The Sacral Chakra governs creativity, sexuality, and emotional balance. Guilt, shame, and unresolved emotional trauma can block this chakra, leading to reproductive and urinary issues, and in extreme cases, cancers of the reproductive organs such as cervical, ovarian, or prostate cancer.

Solar Plexus Chakra (Manipura): The Solar Plexus Chakra is the center of personal power, self-esteem, and confidence. Persistent thoughts of failure, inadequacy, or low self-worth can create blockages here, leading to digestive issues and metabolic disorders, and potentially contributing to the development of stomach or liver cancer.

Heart Chakra (Anahata): The Heart Chakra is the seat of love, compassion, and emotional well-being. Long-term grief, loss, and inability to forgive can block this chakra, leading to heart disease and conditions such as breast cancer or lung cancer.

Throat Chakra (Vishuddha): The Throat Chakra governs communication and self-expression. When individuals are unable to speak their truth or express themselves authentically, this chakra can become blocked, potentially leading to thyroid issues, throat problems, and related cancers.

Third Eye Chakra (Ajna): The Third Eye Chakra is associated with intuition, insight, and spiritual vision. Persistent doubts, lack of clarity, and disconnection from one's intuition can create blockages here, which may manifest as cognitive issues, headaches, or even brain cancer.

Crown Chakra (Sahasrara): The Crown Chakra represents spiritual connection and enlightenment. When this chakra is blocked by feelings of disconnection or spiritual apathy, it can lead to neurological issues and a sense of purposelessness. While not directly associated with specific cancers, an imbalanced Crown Chakra can contribute to an overall state of disease.

The Role of Parasites in Cancerous Thoughts

Parasites are organisms that live on or inside a host, often causing harm. In a spiritual sense, they can be seen as manifestations of negative energy that feed on the individual's life force. Just as physical parasites drain the body's resources, spiritual parasites can exacerbate cancerous thoughts, leading to further physical and emotional deterioration.

Physical Parasites and Energy Blockages: Physical parasites such as worms, flukes, and protozoa can disrupt the body's energy flow by creating inflammation, draining nutrients, and weakening the immune system. This can lead to increased stress and anxiety, which in turn can amplify negative thought patterns and block the chakras.

Metaphorical Parasites: Beyond physical parasites, negative thoughts and emotions themselves can be seen as parasitic, feeding on the individual's energy and leading to further imbalances. These "mental parasites" thrive in environments where there is unresolved trauma, fear, or anger, contributing to the development of disease.

The Connection Between Parasites and Cancer: Chronic parasitic infections have been linked to certain types of cancer. For example, liver flukes have been associated with bile duct cancer, and schistosomes with bladder cancer. These infections create a constant state of inflammation and stress in the body, which can weaken the immune system and make the body more susceptible to cancerous growths.

The Physical Manifestation of Cancerous Thoughts

Cancerous thoughts, when left unchecked, can manifest physically in the body as chronic diseases, including cancer. This manifestation is a result of the prolonged negative impact these thoughts have on the body's energy system, leading to blockages in the chakras, weakening the immune system, and creating an environment where disease can thrive.

Chronic Stress and Disease: Persistent negative thoughts contribute to chronic stress, which is known to be a major risk factor for various diseases. Chronic stress leads to the overproduction of stress hormones like cortisol, which can suppress the immune system, increase inflammation, and alter cellular function—conditions that can contribute to the development of cancer.

Emotional Suppression and Cancer: Emotions that are suppressed or unexpressed—such as anger, grief, or shame—can fester within the body, creating toxic energy that disrupts cellular function. Over time, this toxic energy can contribute to the development of cancer, particularly in organs associated with the blocked chakras.

Case Studies and Scientific Research: While the direct link between negative thoughts and cancer is still a subject of ongoing research, there is increasing evidence to suggest that psychological factors can influence the onset and progression of cancer. Studies have shown that individuals with high levels of stress, unresolved trauma, or chronic negative thinking patterns may have a higher risk of developing cancer.

Healing and Purging Cancerous Thoughts

Healing cancerous thoughts requires a holistic approach that addresses both the mind and body. By identifying and purging these destructive thought patterns, individuals can restore balance to their chakras, strengthen their energy systems, and promote physical healing.

Mindfulness and Meditation: Practices such as mindfulness and meditation can help individuals become aware of their thought patterns and develop the ability to change them. By focusing on positive thoughts and emotions, individuals can counteract the effects of cancerous thoughts and promote healing.

Chakra Balancing: Regular chakra balancing practices, such as yoga, energy healing, and visualization, can help clear blockages and restore the flow of prana throughout the body. This can reduce stress, improve immune function, and create an environment where the body can heal itself.

Detoxification and Parasite Cleansing: Detoxifying the body and clearing physical parasites can help remove the sources of negative energy and reduce the burden on the body's immune system. This can be achieved through dietary changes, herbal cleanses, and other natural remedies.

Therapeutic Practices: Engaging in therapy, whether it be cognitive-behavioral therapy, trauma therapy, or other forms of psychological counseling, can help individuals address the root causes of their cancerous thoughts. By resolving past traumas and learning to reframe negative thought patterns, individuals can break the cycle of negativity and promote overall health.

Conclusion:

The Power of Thought in Shaping Health

The relationship between thoughts and physical health is complex and deeply interconnected. Cancerous thoughts, when left unchecked, can have profound effects on both the mind and body, leading to the development of chronic diseases, including cancer. These thoughts, fueled by fear, guilt, shame, and unresolved emotional trauma, can create energetic blockages in the body, particularly in the chakras. Over time, these blockages disrupt the flow of prana, weaken the immune system, and create an environment conducive to disease.

However, by understanding the origins of cancerous thoughts and their impact on the body's energy system, individuals can take proactive steps to heal and protect themselves. Through mindfulness, meditation, chakra balancing, and other holistic practices, individuals can purge these destructive thoughts and restore balance to their energy systems. By doing so, they not only improve their mental and emotional well-being but also create a foundation for long-term physical health.

The journey to healing from cancerous thoughts is a deeply personal and spiritual one, requiring a commitment to self-awareness, self-care, and spiritual growth. By embracing this journey, individuals can reclaim their power, restore their health, and live in harmony with the divine energy that flows through all life.

Chapter 9

Parasitic Excretions: Hidden Carcinogens and Their Role in Cancer Development

Introduction

The human body is a complex ecosystem where various microorganisms, including parasites, coexist. While some parasites may appear relatively harmless, others can inflict serious harm not just by feeding on their hosts but by releasing toxic excretions. Recent studies suggest that these excretions may act as hidden carcinogens, creating a toxic environment within the body that could potentially lead to cancer. In this chapter, we will explore the fascinating yet dangerous role of parasitic excretions, their impact on the host's body, and how they may contribute to cancer development.

Understanding Parasite Excretions

Parasites come in various forms—helminths (worms), protozoa (single-celled organisms), and ectoparasites (external parasites like lice and ticks). Regardless of their type, many parasites rely on excretion to remove waste products from their bodies. These excretions often contain a cocktail of toxic substances, enzymes, and metabolites that can interfere with the host's cellular environment.

For instance, helminths like the liver fluke (Opisthorchis viverrini) and the bladder fluke (Schistosoma haematobium) release metabolic byproducts that damage tissues and cause inflammation. Over time, this chronic irritation and damage can set the stage for malignant transformations in the host cells, leading to cancers of the bile duct and bladder, respectively. Similarly, protozoan parasites such as Toxoplasma gondii can release enzymes that alter the host's cellular functions, further contributing to a hostile internal environment that is conducive to cancer growth.

The Carcinogenic Pathways of Parasitic Excretions

Parasitic excretions are not merely waste; they are potent biochemical agents that can disrupt normal cellular processes. These excretions often contain free radicals, oxidative agents, and pro-inflammatory molecules. When these toxic substances accumulate in the host's tissues, they can initiate several carcinogenic pathways:

- *Chronic Inflammation: Parasite excretions can cause long-lasting inflammation in the host's body. Inflammation is a well-established risk factor for cancer because it leads to continuous cell damage and regeneration. Each cycle of damage and repair increases the likelihood of DNA mutations that could lead to cancer.*
- *Oxidative Stress: Parasites release reactive oxygen species (ROS) and nitrogen species as part of their metabolic processes. These ROS can damage cellular DNA, proteins, and lipids, leading to mutations and cancerous growths. The body's natural antioxidant defenses may be overwhelmed by the sheer amount of oxidative stress caused by a persistent parasitic infection.*
- *Immune System Modulation: Parasites often manipulate the host's immune system to evade detection. This suppression or alteration of immune responses can create an environment where cancer cells can thrive unnoticed. A suppressed immune system is less capable of identifying and destroying aberrant cells that could potentially turn into tumors.*
- *Direct Cellular Damage: Some parasites, like Schistosoma species, release enzymes that directly damage epithelial cells, leading to cellular dysplasia—a precursor to cancer. Over time, the cumulative effect of this damage can result in malignant transformation.*

Host-Parasite Interaction and Immune Modulation

The relationship between a parasite and its host is complex and dynamic. Parasites are not only adept at evading the host's immune defenses, but they also often suppress them. This suppression allows them to survive within the host, but it also has a secondary effect: it weakens the body's natural ability to fight off not only infections but also cancerous cells.

For example, in the case of helminths like Schistosoma haematobium, the parasite's presence can lead to a Th2-dominated immune response, which suppresses the more aggressive Th1 response that would typically target abnormal cells. This suppression can leave the body vulnerable to both chronic infection and the development of tumors.

Case Studies and Research Evidence

Numerous studies have established a correlation between chronic parasitic infections and cancer:

- *Liver Flukes and Cholangiocarcinoma: The liver fluke, Opisthorchis viverrini, is endemic in parts of Southeast Asia. In regions where this parasite is prevalent, there is a significantly higher incidence of cholangiocarcinoma, a cancer of the bile ducts. Researchers have found that the excretory-secretory products of the parasite can induce DNA damage in host cells, supporting the hypothesis that these excretions are carcinogenic.*
- *Bladder Flukes and Bladder Cancer: In parts of Africa where Schistosoma haematobium infections are common, there is a parallel rise in bladder cancer cases. The parasite's excretions cause chronic inflammation and granuloma formation in the bladder, creating a conducive environment for cancerous growths.*
- *Toxoplasmosis and Brain Tumors: While more research is needed, some studies suggest a possible link between Toxoplasma gondii infections and brain cancers. The parasite's ability to manipulate host cell signaling and immune responses may play a role in tumor development.*

A Holistic Approach to Prevention and Healing

Understanding the connection between parasitic excretions and cancer underscores the importance of a holistic approach to health. It is not enough to merely cleanse the body of parasites; one must also address the underlying conditions—both physical and psychological—that make the body a suitable host. Diet, detoxification, and herbal remedies can play a role in eliminating parasites and neutralizing their toxic byproducts. Equally important is the practice of controlling one's thoughts and emotions, as these too can influence the body's susceptibility to parasitic infestation and disease.

Conclusion

The potential link between parasitic excretions and cancer opens up a new frontier in the understanding of disease. While more research is needed to fully comprehend these connections, the evidence suggests that maintaining a clean internal environment—free from both parasites and negative thoughts—is crucial for holistic health. By understanding and addressing the multifaceted nature of parasitic infections and their toxic excretions, we can take a more comprehensive approach to healing and wellness.

Chapter 10

The Divine Dance of the Senses: A Yogi and Christ Perspective on Awareness and Influence

Introduction: The Harmony of the Senses in Spiritual Awareness

In the vast tapestry of human experience, the senses play a crucial role in shaping our perception of reality. They serve as the gateways through which we interact with the world, influencing our thoughts, emotions, and spiritual well-being. The senses are not merely physical faculties; they are deeply intertwined with our spiritual nature, affecting the balance of our chakras and the flow of prana (life energy) within our bodies. From both a yogic and Christ-centered perspective, understanding the influence of the senses is key to achieving spiritual awareness and maintaining a harmonious existence.

This chapter explores the profound relationship between the senses, chakras, and spiritual awareness, highlighting the consequences of neglecting these aspects of our being. We will delve into the origins and significance of awareness and influence, and how they shape our inner and outer worlds. Additionally, we will examine the deeper meaning behind the saying "Be still and know that I AM God," expanding it to "Be still and know who I AM and that we are all gods," reflecting the divine potential within each individual.

The Five Senses and Their Connection to the Chakras

The five senses—sight, hearing, taste, touch, and smell—are traditionally viewed as the primary means through which we perceive the external world. However, these senses also play a significant role in our internal spiritual experience, influencing the balance of the chakras and the flow of prana within the body.

Sight (Ajna Chakra): The sense of sight is closely connected to the Third Eye Chakra (Ajna), which governs intuition, insight, and spiritual vision. When this chakra is balanced, the individual can perceive reality with clarity and discernment. However, overexposure to negative imagery, such as violence or materialism, can cloud this chakra, leading to confusion, lack of direction, and difficulty accessing one's inner wisdom.

Hearing (Vishuddha Chakra): Hearing is linked to the Throat Chakra (Vishuddha), which is responsible for communication, self-expression, and truth. The sounds we expose ourselves to—whether harmonious or discordant—can either enhance or disrupt the flow of energy in this chakra. Negative auditory stimuli, such as harsh criticism or constant noise, can block the Throat Chakra, leading to difficulties in communication and self-expression.

Taste (Manipura Chakra): The sense of taste is associated with the Solar Plexus Chakra (Manipura), which governs personal power, self-esteem, and digestion. The foods we consume not only affect our physical health but also influence our energetic balance. Consuming unhealthy or impure foods can disrupt the Solar Plexus Chakra, leading to issues related to self-worth, confidence, and digestive health.

Touch (Anahata Chakra): Touch is connected to the Heart Chakra (Anahata), the center of love, compassion, and emotional balance. Positive physical contact, such as hugging or holding hands, can open and heal the Heart Chakra. Conversely, negative or abusive touch can block this chakra, causing emotional wounds and difficulties in forming healthy relationships.

Smell (Muladhara Chakra): The sense of smell is linked to the Root Chakra (Muladhara), which is the foundation of our survival instincts and grounding. The aromas we encounter can have a powerful impact on this chakra. Pleasant, grounding scents, such as those from nature, can strengthen the Root Chakra, while foul odors or toxic fumes can weaken it, leading to feelings of insecurity and fear.

The Concept of Awareness

Awareness is the state of being conscious of one's surroundings, thoughts, emotions, and inner state. It is the foundation of spiritual growth, enabling individuals to recognize and address the influences that shape their lives. The concept of awareness is central to many spiritual traditions, including both yoga and Christianity.

Origins of Awareness in Spiritual Traditions: In yoga, awareness is cultivated through practices such as meditation, pranayama, and asana (physical postures). These practices help individuals develop a heightened sense of self-awareness, enabling them to observe their thoughts, emotions, and bodily sensations without attachment. In Christianity, awareness is often associated with the concept of mindfulness and the practice of prayer, where individuals seek to align themselves with God's will and remain conscious of His presence in their lives.

Awareness and the Senses: Awareness of the senses is crucial for maintaining the balance of the chakras and the flow of prana within the body. By becoming aware of the sensory stimuli we are exposed to, we can make conscious choices that support our spiritual and physical well-being. For example, choosing to listen to uplifting music, eat nourishing foods, and engage in positive physical contact can enhance our energy levels and promote a sense of inner peace.

The Role of Awareness in Healing: Awareness is also a powerful tool for healing. By becoming aware of the negative thoughts, emotions, and behaviors that contribute to disease, individuals can begin to address and transform these patterns. This process is essential for purging cancerous thoughts and restoring balance to the chakras, ultimately leading to physical and spiritual healing.

The Concept of Influence

Influence refers to the capacity to have an effect on the character, development, or behavior of someone or something. In the context of spirituality, influence can be understood as the impact that external stimuli—such as sensory experiences, environmental factors, and social interactions—have on an individual's inner state.

Origins of Influence in Spiritual Traditions: The concept of influence is deeply rooted in both Eastern and Western spiritual traditions. In yoga, the idea of influence is closely related to the concept of samskaras (impressions or imprints left by past actions and experiences) and how they shape an individual's karma and spiritual path. In Christianity, influence is often discussed in terms of temptation, sin, and the importance of surrounding oneself with positive influences that align with God's will.

The Influence of the Senses on the Chakras: The senses have a profound influence on the chakras, as the stimuli they receive can either support or disrupt the flow of energy within the body. For example, consuming unhealthy food can negatively affect the Solar Plexus Chakra, leading to digestive issues and a loss of personal power. Similarly, exposure to negative sounds can block the Throat Chakra, impairing communication and self-expression.

Managing Influence for Spiritual Growth: To cultivate spiritual growth, it is essential to manage the influences we allow into our lives. This involves being mindful of the sensory stimuli we are exposed to and making conscious choices that support our well-being. For example, choosing to spend time in nature, engage in positive social interactions, and practice mindfulness can help maintain the balance of the chakras and promote spiritual awareness.

he Negative Side of Neglect

Neglecting the senses and their influence on our spiritual and physical health can have serious consequences. When we are not mindful of the sensory stimuli we expose ourselves to, we can become overwhelmed by negative influences, leading to energetic imbalances and disease.

Energetic Imbalances and Disease: When the chakras are blocked or imbalanced due to negative sensory influences, the flow of prana within the body is disrupted. This can lead to physical and emotional ailments, including chronic stress, anxiety, depression, and disease. For example, neglecting the sense of taste by consuming unhealthy foods can disrupt the Solar Plexus Chakra, leading to digestive issues and a loss of personal power.

Cancerous Thoughts and Physical Manifestation: Persistent exposure to negative sensory stimuli can also lead to the development of cancerous thoughts, which can manifest physically as disease. For example, constant exposure to negative media or toxic environments can create a state of chronic stress, which weakens the immune system and increases the risk of developing cancer. By neglecting the importance of sensory awareness, we open ourselves up to these destructive influences.

The Importance of Mindfulness and Discipline: To avoid the negative consequences of neglect, it is essential to practice mindfulness and discipline in our daily lives. This involves being aware of the sensory stimuli we encounter and making conscious choices that support our well-being. By cultivating a disciplined approach to our senses, we can maintain the balance of the chakras, promote spiritual growth, and prevent the development of disease.

Be Still and Know Who I AM

The phrase "Be still and know that I AM God" is a powerful reminder of the importance of stillness and inner reflection in spiritual practice. However, this phrase can be expanded to reflect a deeper understanding of our divine nature: "Be still and know who I AM and that we are all gods."

The Deeper Meaning of Stillness: Stillness is not just the absence of movement; it is a state of inner peace and awareness. In this state, we can connect with our true selves and recognize our divine nature. By being still, we can tune out the distractions of the external world and listen to the voice of God within us.

Recognizing Our Divine Nature: The expanded phrase "Be still and know who I AM and that we are all gods" reflects the belief that each individual possesses a spark of the divine. In both yogic and Christian traditions, this idea is expressed in different ways. In yoga, it is believed that the soul (Atman) is a reflection of the universal consciousness (Brahman). In Christianity, humans are made in the image of God, and through Christ, we are called to realize our divine potential.

The Power of Self-Realization: By recognizing our divine nature, we can begin to take responsibility for our thoughts, actions, and the influences we allow into our lives. This self-realization empowers us to make conscious choices that support our spiritual growth and well-being. It is through this awareness that we can fully embody our potential as co-creators of our reality, aligning our will with the divine purpose.

The Role of Stillness in Spiritual Practice: Stillness, both physical and mental, is a key practice in both yoga and Christianity. In yoga, meditation serves as a means to quiet the mind, allowing for a deeper connection with the self and the divine. In Christianity, stillness is often associated with prayer and contemplation, creating space for communion with God. In both traditions, stillness is seen as essential for developing spiritual awareness and insight.

The Divine Nature of All Beings: Expanding the phrase to "Be still and know who I AM and that we are all gods" also emphasizes the interconnectedness of all beings. In recognizing our own divinity, we must also acknowledge the divine spark in others. This recognition fosters compassion, empathy, and a sense of unity, which are crucial for spiritual growth and harmonious living.

The Interplay Between the Senses, Chakras, and Cancerous Thoughts

The senses are deeply intertwined with the chakras and the overall energetic balance within the body. When the senses are overwhelmed or neglected, they can contribute to the development of cancerous thoughts—negative thought patterns that, like a physical malignancy, can spread and cause harm.

How Senses Influence Chakras: Each sense is connected to specific chakras, and the stimuli we receive through these senses can either support or disrupt the flow of energy. For example, visual stimuli that are uplifting and positive can enhance the balance of the Third Eye Chakra, promoting clarity and insight. Conversely, exposure to negative or violent imagery can create blockages, leading to confusion and mental distress.

Cancerous Thoughts as Energetic Blockages: Persistent negative thoughts are like energetic blockages within the body. They disrupt the natural flow of prana, creating imbalances that can manifest as physical ailments. These cancerous thoughts are often reinforced by negative sensory experiences, which feed the cycle of negativity and disease.

The Role of Awareness in Preventing Disease: Awareness of the senses and their influence on the chakras is essential for preventing the development of cancerous thoughts and their physical manifestations. By cultivating awareness, individuals can make conscious choices about the stimuli they expose themselves to, thereby supporting their energetic balance and overall health.

Practical Strategies for Cultivating Awareness and Influence

To harness the power of awareness and influence in daily life, it is important to adopt practices that support the balance of the chakras and the positive engagement of the senses.

Mindful Consumption of Sensory Stimuli: Be selective about the sensory experiences you engage with. Choose media, environments, and interactions that uplift and inspire, rather than those that drain or distress. For example, spend time in nature, listen to soothing music, and surround yourself with positive influences.

Chakra Meditation and Balancing: Regularly practice chakra meditation to clear blockages and restore balance to your energy centers. Focus on each chakra in turn, using visualization, affirmations, and breathwork to enhance the flow of prana. This practice can help you maintain a clear mind and a healthy body.

Integrating Stillness into Daily Life: Incorporate moments of stillness and reflection into your daily routine. Whether through meditation, prayer, or simply taking a few deep breaths, these moments allow you to reconnect with your inner self and the divine. Use this time to reflect on your thoughts, feelings, and sensory experiences, and to align yourself with your higher purpose.

Conscious Living and Decision-Making: Make conscious choices about the influences you allow into your life. Consider how your actions, environment, and interactions affect your spiritual and *physical health. By living consciously, you can take control of your life's direction, ensuring that you are guided by positive influences that support your growth.*

The Consequences of Neglect and the Path to Healing

Neglecting the importance of sensory awareness and the influence of the chakras can lead to a range of negative consequences, both physically and spiritually. However, by recognizing and addressing these issues, it is possible to reverse their effects and embark on a path to healing.

The Impact of Neglect on Health: When sensory awareness is neglected, and negative influences are allowed to dominate, the chakras become imbalanced, and the flow of prana is disrupted. This can lead to a host of physical and emotional problems, including chronic stress, anxiety, depression, and even diseases such as cancer.

Reversing the Effects of Neglect: Healing begins with awareness. By becoming aware of the negative influences in your life, you can take steps to eliminate them and replace them with positive, life-affirming experiences. This process involves purging cancerous thoughts, detoxifying the body and mind, and restoring balance to the chakras.

The Path to Spiritual Healing: Spiritual healing requires a commitment to self-awareness, self-care, and spiritual practice. By embracing practices such as mindfulness, meditation, chakra balancing, and positive sensory engagement, you can heal from the effects of neglect and cultivate a deep sense of inner peace and spiritual fulfillment.

Conclusion:

Embracing the Divine Dance of the Senses

The senses are a divine gift, allowing us to experience the world in all its richness and complexity. However, they must be engaged with awareness and discernment to maintain the balance of our chakras and the flow of prana within our bodies. By understanding the interplay between the senses, chakras, and thoughts, we can harness their power to promote spiritual growth, physical health, and emotional well-being.

The expanded understanding of the phrase "Be still and know who I AM and that we are all gods" reflects the profound potential within each of us to live a life of awareness, influence, and divine connection. By cultivating stillness, awareness, and conscious living, we can align ourselves with our true nature and realize our divine potential.

This chapter has provided a deep exploration of the role of the senses, awareness, and influence in spiritual and physical health. It emphasizes the importance of mindful engagement with the senses, the consequences of neglect, and the path to healing through self-awareness and spiritual practice. By embracing these principles, we can live a life that is harmonious, balanced, and in alignment with the divine.

Chapter 11

The Alchemy of Breath and CSF Circulation: A Deep Exploration of Mindful Meditation and Neurophysiology

Introduction: The Intersection of Mind, Breath, and Body

In the pursuit of spiritual awakening and physical health, the practice of mindful meditation has long been recognized as a powerful tool. However, the profound effects of breathwork and meditation extend beyond the mind, influencing the body's most intricate systems, including the circulation of cerebrospinal fluid (CSF). This chapter explores the deep connection between mindful meditation, breath control, and the movement of CSF, offering a comprehensive understanding of how these practices promote both spiritual and physical well-being.

By merging the wisdom of ancient yogic traditions with modern scientific insights, we will delve into the alchemy of breath—the transformative power of controlled breathing—and its role in enhancing CSF circulation and overall neurological health. This chapter aims to provide a clear yet profound explanation of these concepts, emphasizing the importance of integrating mindful meditation into daily life.

The Alchemy of Breath—Transforming Consciousness

Breath is the bridge between the body and the mind. It is a powerful tool that can be harnessed to influence our physical, emotional, and spiritual states. In yogic traditions, breath control, or pranayama, is considered essential for achieving higher states of consciousness and maintaining physical health.

Pranayama: The Science of Breath: Pranayama, derived from the Sanskrit words "prana" (life force) and "ayama" (extension), refers to the practice of controlling the breath to expand and direct the flow of prana within the body. Various pranayama techniques, such as alternate nostril breathing (Nadi Shodhana) and breath retention (Kumbhaka), are designed to balance the energy systems, calm the mind, and prepare the practitioner for deeper meditation.

Breath as a Tool for Mindfulness: In mindfulness meditation, the breath serves as an anchor for attention, helping practitioners cultivate present-moment awareness. By focusing on the rhythm of the breath, individuals can quiet the mental chatter and achieve a state of inner stillness. This practice not only enhances mental clarity but also has profound effects on the body's physiology.

The Physiological Effects of Controlled Breathing: Controlled breathing has been shown to influence the autonomic nervous system, promoting relaxation and reducing stress. It activates the parasympathetic nervous system, which is responsible for the "rest and digest" response, leading to lower heart rates, reduced blood pressure, and improved digestion. These physiological changes create an optimal environment for the circulation of CSF, which plays a crucial role in maintaining neurological health.

Cerebrospinal Fluid—The Elixir of the Nervous System

Cerebrospinal fluid (CSF) is a clear, colorless fluid that surrounds the brain and spinal cord, providing protection, nourishment, and waste removal. It is often referred to as the "elixir" of the nervous system due to its vital role in maintaining brain health and function.

The Production and Circulation of CSF: CSF is produced primarily in the choroid plexus of the brain's ventricles. It circulates through the ventricles, around the brain and spinal cord, and is eventually reabsorbed into the bloodstream. This circulation is essential for cushioning the brain, maintaining stable pressure within the skull, and removing metabolic waste products from the central nervous system.

The Role of CSF in Brain Health: CSF plays a critical role in maintaining the brain's environment, ensuring that neurons function optimally. It helps regulate the brain's extracellular fluid, supports neurotransmitter balance, and provides a medium for the exchange of nutrients and waste. Disruptions in CSF circulation have been linked to neurological disorders, such as hydrocephalus, where excess CSF causes increased pressure on the brain.

CSF and Spiritual Traditions: In various spiritual traditions, the movement of CSF is linked to the awakening of higher consciousness. The ancient yogis believed that the flow of prana through the spinal cord, facilitated by breath control, could enhance the circulation of CSF, leading to spiritual enlightenment. This concept is mirrored in modern practices that emphasize the importance of spinal health and the alignment of energy centers, or chakras, in achieving spiritual awakening.

The Connection Between Breath, Meditation, and CSF Circulation

The relationship between breath control, meditation, and CSF circulation is profound. Through specific techniques, individuals can influence the movement of CSF, enhancing its ability to nourish and protect the brain while promoting spiritual awareness.

Breath Control and CSF Movement: Certain breathing techniques, particularly those involving breath retention and rhythmic patterns, create gentle pressure changes within the thoracic cavity and the spinal column. These pressure changes can facilitate the movement of CSF, encouraging its circulation throughout the brain and spinal cord. This enhanced circulation is believed to support the removal of toxins, improve nutrient delivery to neurons, and promote overall brain health.

Meditation and the Spinal Column: During meditation, especially when combined with breath control, the focus is often directed toward the spine, which is seen as the central channel for energy flow (Sushumna Nadi in yogic terms). This focus helps to align the vertebrae and create an optimal environment for CSF circulation. The stillness achieved in meditation further supports the gentle movement of CSF, enhancing its protective and nourishing functions.

The Role of Vibration and Sound: In addition to breath control, sound and vibration can influence CSF circulation. Chanting, humming, or listening to specific frequencies can create resonant vibrations that travel through the body, including the spinal column. These vibrations can stimulate the movement of CSF, enhance the flow of prana, and promote a state of deep relaxation and spiritual connection.

The Impact of Neglecting Breath and CSF Health

Neglecting the practice of mindful breathing and the health of CSF can lead to a range of physical, mental, and spiritual issues. When breath becomes shallow or irregular, and when CSF circulation is disrupted, the body's natural balance is compromised, leading to various health problems.

Consequences of Shallow Breathing: Shallow, rapid breathing is a common response to stress and anxiety, but it can have detrimental effects on the body. It can lead to hyperventilation, decreased oxygen levels in the blood, and an imbalance in carbon dioxide levels. This disrupts the autonomic nervous system and can contribute to chronic stress, anxiety, and fatigue. Over time, it can also impair CSF circulation, reducing its ability to protect and nourish the brain.

Impaired CSF Circulation: When CSF circulation is impaired, the brain's ability to maintain a stable internal environment is compromised. This can lead to increased intracranial pressure, impaired waste removal, and the buildup of toxins in the brain. Such conditions are associated with neurological disorders, cognitive decline, and an increased risk of diseases such as Alzheimer's.

Spiritual Stagnation: On a spiritual level, neglecting breath control and CSF health can lead to a sense of stagnation, disconnection, and a lack of spiritual progress. The flow of prana becomes restricted, and the chakras may become blocked, preventing the individual from achieving higher states of consciousness and spiritual awareness.

Integrating Mindful Breathing and CSF Health into Daily Life

To support both physical and spiritual health, it is essential to integrate mindful breathing practices and techniques that promote healthy CSF circulation into daily life. By doing so, individuals can enhance their well-being, protect their brain health, and deepen their spiritual practice.

Daily Breathwork Practices: Incorporate pranayama techniques into your daily routine. Begin with simple practices, such as deep diaphragmatic breathing, and gradually introduce more advanced techniques like alternate nostril breathing or breath retention. Consistent practice will help regulate your nervous system, improve oxygenation, and support the movement of CSF.

Meditation and Spinal Alignment: During meditation, pay attention to your posture, ensuring that your spine is aligned and your head is balanced atop your neck. This alignment supports the natural movement of CSF and the flow of energy through the chakras. Consider using a meditation cushion or chair to help maintain proper alignment.

Incorporating Sound and Vibration: Use sound and vibration to enhance your meditation and breathwork practices. Chanting mantras, humming, or listening to specific frequencies can stimulate the movement of CSF and deepen your connection to the divine. Experiment with different sounds to find what resonates with you.

Physical Movement and Spinal Health: Regular physical activity, particularly exercises that promote spinal flexibility and strength, can support CSF circulation. Yoga, tai chi, and Pilates are excellent practices for maintaining spinal health and encouraging the flow of prana and CSF.

Conclusion:

The Synergy of Breath and CSF in Spiritual and Physical Health

The alchemy of breath, as explored through the lens of ancient yogic traditions and modern scientific understanding, reveals the profound impact that controlled breathing can have on both the mind and body. Through the practice of pranayama, meditation, and mindful awareness, individuals can influence the movement of cerebrospinal fluid, enhance their mental clarity, and promote overall well-being.

By integrating these practices into daily life, we can harness the power of breath to support the natural circulation of CSF, ensuring that our brain and spinal cord are nourished, protected, and free from toxins. This holistic approach to health emphasizes the importance of maintaining balance in both the physical and spiritual realms, recognizing that true well-being is achieved when the mind, body, and spirit are in harmony.

Furthermore, this chapter has highlighted the importance of spinal alignment, sound, and vibration in enhancing the movement of CSF and supporting the flow of prana through the chakras. These practices not only contribute to physical health but also facilitate spiritual awakening, allowing individuals to access higher states of consciousness and deepen their connection with the divine.

In summary, the integration of mindful breathing and CSF circulation practices offers a powerful means of achieving holistic health. By embracing these practices, we can cultivate a deep sense of inner peace, protect our neurological health, and embark on a journey of spiritual growth. This chapter serves as a guide to understanding the profound connection between breath, CSF, and spiritual awareness, providing a foundation for a life of harmony, balance, and fulfillment.

Chapter 12

Mindfulness Meditation and Breath Control

This practice is a form of mindfulness meditation combined with breath control, which has profound effects on both the neurological and physiological levels.

Here's a breakdown of what you will be doing and the effects it has:

1. Counting Backward and Focusing on Breath

What You're Doing: *Counting backward from 180 to 0 while focusing on your breath helps to anchor your mind in the present moment. This practice can reduce mental chatter and enhance concentration.*

Neurological Effects: *This activates the prefrontal cortex, which is involved in attention and cognitive control. The simple act of counting, combined with breath awareness, promotes the engagement of the parasympathetic nervous system, leading to a state of calm and relaxation. The repetitive nature of the counting helps to quiet the default mode network (DMN), which is often active during mind-wandering and is associated with self-referential thoughts.*

2. Controlled Breathing (4-Second Inhale, 6-Second Exhale)

What You're Doing: *By controlling the rhythm of your breathing, you're engaging in what is often referred to as paced breathing. The specific 4:6 ratio is slightly elongated on the exhale, which is known to enhance relaxation.*

Neurological Effects: *This practice stimulates the vagus nerve, which plays a key role in regulating the parasympathetic nervous system. The longer exhalation activates the vagus nerve more effectively, leading to a reduction in heart rate variability and promoting a state of rest and digestion. This can also reduce the production of stress hormones like cortisol while increasing GABA, a neurotransmitter that has calming effects on the brain.*

3. Chakra-Focused Breathing

What You're Doing: *Directing your breath through each chakra while maintaining the controlled breathing pattern.*

Neurological Effects: While the concept of chakras is more spiritual, focusing on different areas of the body during breathwork can be likened to body scanning in mindfulness meditation. This increases interoception, the ability to sense internal body states, which is linked to enhanced emotional regulation and self-awareness. The sequential focus on different parts of the body can also help to balance the autonomic nervous system, creating a more harmonious state of mind and body.

4. Breathing Through the Entire Body

What You're Doing: After focusing on each chakra, you shift your attention to the entire body, maintaining the breathing rhythm.

Neurological Effects: This broader focus likely promotes a state of whole-body awareness, which can lead to a profound sense of unity and presence. Engaging the entire body in your awareness can enhance the overall connectivity within the brain, particularly between regions involved in sensory processing, emotional regulation, and executive function. It also deepens the relaxation response, potentially inducing states of flow or even altered states of consciousness where you experience a sense of oneness with your surroundings.

Why These Effects Occur:

Brain Plasticity: Regular practice of such meditation and breathwork promotes neuroplasticity, the brain's ability to reorganize itself by forming new neural connections. This can improve emotional resilience, cognitive function, and overall mental well-being.

Stress Reduction: The reduction of activity in the DMN, combined with the activation of the parasympathetic nervous system, leads to a significant reduction in stress and anxiety. This is accompanied by physiological benefits, such as lowered blood pressure and improved immune function.

In summary, this meditation practice is a powerful method for promoting mental clarity, emotional stability, and physical relaxation, all of which contribute to overall well-being.

A Guided Meditation

Begin with Stillness

Sit with a straight spine, rooted in the earth, and allow your body to come to rest. Close your eyes gently, as if you are embracing the darkness within. In this stillness, you are like the mountain, unmovable, yet alive with the energy of the earth beneath you.

Observe the Mind's Nature

Some days, the mind will be calm, like a tranquil lake, reflecting the sky above. On other days, thoughts will flutter like restless birds, and your mind may seem like a stormy sea. Do not judge these fluctuations. Simply observe them as the natural flow of the mind. If the thoughts are many, do not fight them. Instead, use a gentle tool: begin to count backward from 180 to 0.

Anchor Yourself in the Breath

As you count, draw your attention to the breath. Feel the coolness of the inhale, like a breeze entering a shaded forest. Feel the warmth of the exhale, as though the breath is a stream of warmth flowing from the depths of your being. Let this awareness of the breath become your anchor, steadying your mind as you count.

Transition to Controlled Breathing

When you reach zero, pause in the stillness you have cultivated. Now, begin to guide your breath more consciously. Inhale to the count of four, the life force, and exhale to the count of six, releasing all tension and stress. Allow the breath to flow smoothly, like a river, neither rushing nor hesitating.

Focus on the Chakras

Once the breath has found its 4:6 breath cycle, direct your attention to the base of your spine, to the Root Chakra. With each inhale and with each exhale, imagine drawing energy through the area at the base of the spine. Breathe three times here.

Then, gently move your awareness upward to the Sacral Chakra, located just below your navel. With each inhale and with each exhale, imagine drawing energy through the area below the navel. Breathe three times here.

Next, shift your focus to the Solar Plexus Chakra, just above your navel. With each inhale and with each exhale, imagine drawing energy through the area above the navel. Breathe three times here.

Move now to the Heart Chakra, at the center of your chest. Let the breath open your heart, with each inhale and with each exhale, imagine drawing energy through the heart area. Breathe three times here.

Then, focus on the Throat Chakra, at the base of your throat. With each inhale and with each exhale, imagine drawing energy through the throat area. Breathe three times here.

Bring your attention now to the Third Eye Chakra, between your eyebrows. Let the breath sharpen your inner vision, awakening your intuition. With each inhale and with each exhale, imagine drawing energy through the area between the eyebrows. Breathe three times here.

Finally, rise to the Crown Chakra, at the top of your head. As you breathe, feel a connection to the divine, to the infinite. With each inhale and with each exhale, imagine drawing energy through the top of your head area. Breathe three times here.

Expand to the Whole Body

Now, expand your awareness beyond the chakras. Imagine the breath flowing through your entire body, from the soles of your feet to the crown of your head. Feel your whole being alive with the rhythm of the breath. Maintain the 4:6 breath cycle, allowing this wave of energy to cleanse and unify your entire self.

Rest in Stillness

When you are ready, allow the breath to return to its natural rhythm. Rest in the stillness you have created, feeling the harmony within. Remember, this practice is a journey, not a destination. Each breath, each moment, brings you closer to the divine essence within you.

Conclusion: Integrating the Practice

This practice is more than just a meditation; it is a way to harmonize your physical, mental, and spiritual selves. By aligning with your breath and the chakras, you open the door to inner peace, clarity, and connection with the universe. Continue to practice, with patience and dedication, and you will see the profound transformation it brings to your life.

My Faith in Christ

Introduction:

A Personal Journey of Faith

Faith is a deeply personal journey, shaped by individual experiences, beliefs, and understandings. For me, faith in Christ is not just a religious obligation but a conscious choice to live in alignment with divine truth and love. This chapter explores my understanding of God, Christ, Jesus, and His teachings, and how these elements form the foundation of my spiritual life. It is a reflection of my commitment to live in the Christ, embracing a holistic and spiritual understanding of the world that transcends mere religious rituals.

Understanding God: The Divine Source of All

To me, God is not confined to a singular image or form. God is the divine source of all that exists, encompassing everything within and beyond the physical universe. God is omnipresent, omnipotent, and omniscient, existing in every atom, every thought, and every heartbeat. This understanding aligns with the belief that God is not a man but rather an infinite, formless presence that permeates all of creation.

God's presence is felt in the stillness of meditation, the beauty of nature, and the love shared between beings. God is the life force that animates all living things, the essence of the universe, and the ultimate reality that we all seek to connect with. This understanding of God moves beyond traditional anthropomorphic depictions, offering a more expansive view that resonates with the infinite nature of the divine.

Christ: The Divine Consciousness

When I speak of Christ, I refer to the divine consciousness that exists within all beings—a consciousness that embodies unconditional love, compassion, wisdom, and spiritual understanding. Christ is not limited to the person of Jesus; rather, Christ represents the divine potential within each of us, the part of our being that is eternally connected to God.

Living in Christ means aligning oneself with this divine consciousness, choosing love over fear, compassion over judgment, and truth over deception. It is a commitment to live a life guided by *the principles of Christ-consciousness, which are rooted in the highest expressions of love, kindness, and spiritual awareness.*

Jesus: The Embodiment of Christ-Consciousness

Jesus of Nazareth, whom many know as Jesus Christ, was a profound spiritual teacher and healer who fully embodied Christ-consciousness. His life and teachings provide a blueprint for living in alignment with divine truth and love. Jesus taught that the kingdom of God is within us, that we are all children of God, and that love is the greatest commandment.

Jesus' message was one of inclusivity, compassion, and spiritual liberation. He sought to free people from the chains of fear, guilt, and ignorance, encouraging them to realize their inherent divinity. His teachings on love, forgiveness, and humility are timeless and continue to resonate with those seeking spiritual truth.

Love: The Core of Jesus' Teachings

At the heart of Jesus' teachings is the concept of love—love for God, love for oneself, and love for others. Jesus emphasized that love is the fulfillment of the law and that true spirituality is measured by one's capacity to love unconditionally. This love is not limited to personal affection but extends to all beings, including those who may be difficult to love.

In my understanding, love is the highest vibration, the purest expression of divine consciousness. To live in Christ is to live a life centered on love, striving to embody the love that Jesus taught and demonstrated. This love is not passive; it is an active force that heals, uplifts, and transforms.

Spiritual Understanding: Seeing Beyond the Physical

Spiritual understanding is the ability to see beyond the physical world and recognize the deeper truths that govern our existence. Jesus often spoke in parables, using metaphors and stories to convey spiritual truths that transcend the material realm. He taught that true wealth is not found in earthly possessions but in spiritual treasures, and that the way to eternal life is through spiritual rebirth.

My faith in Christ includes this spiritual understanding—a recognition that we are spiritual beings having a human experience. It involves looking beyond appearances and understanding the spiritual lessons behind life's challenges. This perspective allows me to approach life with a sense of purpose, knowing that every experience is an opportunity for spiritual growth.

Holistic Understanding: Integrating Mind, Body, and Spirit

Holistic understanding involves seeing the interconnectedness of all aspects of life—mind, body, and spirit. Jesus' teachings were not just spiritual but also practical, addressing the needs of the whole person. He healed the sick, fed the hungry, and comforted the brokenhearted, demonstrating that true spirituality encompasses all aspects of life.

Living in Christ means embracing a holistic approach to health and well-being. It involves caring for the body as a temple of the Holy Spirit, nurturing the mind with positive and uplifting thoughts, and nourishing the spirit through prayer, meditation, and acts of kindness. This holistic approach is essential for living a balanced and fulfilled life, one that is in harmony with God's will.

Choosing to Live in the Christ

Choosing to live in Christ is a daily commitment to align my thoughts, actions, and intentions with the divine consciousness that Jesus embodied. It is a conscious choice to live a life of love, compassion, and spiritual awareness, guided by the teachings of Jesus and the principles of Christ-consciousness.

This choice is not always easy, as it requires constant self-reflection, discipline, and a willingness to let go of ego-driven desires. However, the rewards are profound—a deep sense of peace, purpose, and connection ith God. Living in Christ is not about adhering to dogma or rituals; it is about embodying the spirit of Christ in every aspect of life, recognizing that we are all expressions of the divine.

Conclusion:

My Faith, My Path

My faith in Christ is the foundation of my life, guiding me on a path of spiritual growth, holistic health, and deep inner peace. It is a faith that transcends religious boundaries, embracing the universal truths that Jesus taught and lived. By choosing to live in Christ, I am committing to a life of love, compassion, and spiritual awareness, knowing that this is the path that leads to true fulfillment and eternal connection with God.

This chapter is a reflection of my personal understanding of God, Christ, and Jesus, and the profound impact these beliefs have on my life. It is my hope that by sharing my faith, others may be inspired to explore their own spiritual paths and discover the divine potential within themselves.

Disclaimer:

This book, "The Cancer Connection: What They Don't Want You to Know About Parasites, Thoughts, and Healing," presents a unique blend of spiritual, holistic, and speculative perspectives. The ideas and interpretations shared within these pages are the result of the author's reflections, beliefs, and creative exploration, influenced by various spiritual, historical, and contemporary practices and sources.

Readers are encouraged to approach the content with an open mind and discernment. This book is not intended to replace professional medical or mental health guidance. Any practices or suggestions discussed should be considered supplementary and used in conjunction with advice from qualified professionals.

The author acknowledges that healing and health are deeply personal journeys and encourages all readers to seek their own path to well-being.

About the Author:

C. Rice

C. Rice was born on April 22nd, 1971, at 2:30 P.M. in Houston, Texas. His life journey has been anything but ordinary, marked by significant challenges and profound transformations. Having spent the better part of a decade behind bars, C. Rice was last released in March 2010, determined to rebuild his life with a newfound sense of purpose and direction.

During his time in incarceration, C. Rice began a deep spiritual journey that would redefine his understanding of life, faith, and the power of the human mind. Upon his release, he committed himself to a rigorous spiritual practice, reading the Bible in its entirety once a year—a discipline that has led him to complete the sacred text 13 times. This dedication has provided him with a rich foundation of spiritual knowledge and insight, deeply influencing his perspective on life and his approach to spiritual healing.

C. Rice's spiritual practice extends beyond mere reading; he engages daily in a meditative method that he shares in this book. This practice, which he has honed over the years, involves deep mindfulness, breath control, and chakra-focused meditation. For anywhere from 30 minutes to two hours each day, C. Rice immerses himself in this meditative discipline, seeking to align his mind, body, and spirit with the divine energy that flows through all creation.

His life experiences—both the struggles and the triumphs—have given C. Rice a unique perspective on faith, spirituality, and the human condition. His journey from darkness to light, from confinement to liberation, is a testament to the transformative power of faith and the resilience of the human spirit.

In this book, C. Rice brings together his years of spiritual study, personal reflection, and disciplined practice to offer readers a holistic approach to health and spiritual well-being. His teachings are not just theoretical; they are lived experiences, tested and proven through years of dedicated practice. C. Rice's work is a call to awaken to the divine potential within each of us, to live a life of purpose, love, and spiritual awareness.